The
HOLISTIC
DOCTOR

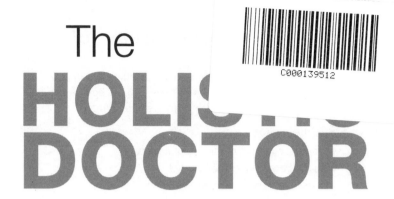

Your guide to
ultimate health
and **wellbeing**

DR DEBORAH McMANNERS

PIATKUS

Copyright © 2004 by Dr Deborah McManners

First published in Great Britain in 2004 by
Piatkus Books Ltd
5 Windmill Street, London W1T 2JA
email: info@piatkus.co.uk

The moral right of the author has been asserted

A catalogue record for this book is available from the British Library

ISBN 0 7499 2440 3

Text design by Paul Saunders
Edited by Barbara Kiser
Illustrations by Lesley Wakerley

This book has been printed on paper manufactured
with respect for the environment using wood from
managed sustainable resources

Typesetting by Palimpsest Book Production Limited,
Polmont, Stirlingshire
Printed and bound in Great Britain by
MPG Books Ltd, Bodmin, Cornwall

Contents

Acknowledgements

My particular and heart-felt thanks go to Karen Evennett, who helped with the later stages of the book. She has been a delight to work with.

It has also been a delight to work with Anna Crago from Piatkus Books, whose advice has been invaluable. I'm also very grateful to Joel Levy, who provided lots of help in the early days, Barbara Kiser, who edited the final draft, and David Eldridge for the splendid jacket design.

I'd like to thank all my patients – all those who have allowed me to use their stories in the book, many of whom urged me to write this book, and not to mention the many others we didn't have room for.

I also wish to thank Judy Piatkus for encouraging me to translate the ideas and experiences of my medical practice into the world of books, to allow me to share what I do with my patients with so many more people. I am also hugely indebted to commissioning editor Gill Bailey, whose perception and persistence pushed us from a set of rather amorphous but exciting ideas, to the clarity and apparent simplicity of the finished article. Thank you both for your much-appreciated help.

One person has been with this project right from when it was just an idea in my own head – my literary agent Barbara Levy, to whom I am most grateful for all manner of vital interventions.

Introduction

In the days before blood tests, scans, and all the diagnostic magic of modern medicine, all physicians were naturopaths, relying upon their own instincts and intuition. With only a few drugs and natural remedies, their job was to create the conditions in which their patients' own internal healing powers could flourish. They used natural treatments like warm springs and cold water, massage, meditation and carefully chosen foods.

Now science teaches us to focus on specific symptoms to which we can apply tried and tested remedies. But humans are very complicated beings, and most medical problems have a psychological dimension too. The original physicians had to look carefully at every aspect of a patient's life and circumstances (if only because they could not order up a battery of lab tests to give them specific answers) – and naturopathy still does this. It recognises an important need: being in harmony with our environment. And it acknowledges that, when harmony is achieved, good health is its attendant.

These days, people know little about that kind of harmony. We push ourselves to emotional exhaustion, but fail to realise that stress and other emotional factors can have a bearing on our physical health. Poor diet and a lack of physical fitness (often with the added problems of smoking and excessive alcohol), have also left many in constant poor health, suffering one illness after another.

As doctors, we are trying to educate people so they can extract themselves from what easily becomes a downward spiral into chronic ill health. But hard-pressed family practitioners – and I am one of them – are often too busy fire-fighting illness and diagnosing disease.

Being happy and healthy has to be a journey that you make for yourself – but you need a map and a compass to help you reach your destination, and, in this book, I hope to give you these basics. I am going to help you to do the very fundamental things that a lot of my patients have lost the ability to do: to understand and listen to your body; to recognise when it is working well, and when it is not; and to give it all the ingredients it needs to flourish and maintain excellent health: the best possible diet, a nourishing environment, optimum physical fitness, and well-deserved rest and relaxation.

After I've introduced you to my methods and practice in Part 1, I'll discuss your health in the way I would in my clinic with patients. I have a lengthy questionnaire that I use, asking patients to tell me about the relevant aspects of their lives – from diet and exercise to physical environment, emotional wellbeing and beyond, so that I can work out how to best help them. In this book I've provided sections of my questionnaire, so that you can learn to look at your own health in the same way that I do.

You'll find parts of the questionnaire throughout the book – you'll be able to see them easily as there'll be a shaded bar down the side wherever they appear. Under a main heading, there'll be a short list of questions. I'd like you to think about your answers to those questions. You may not know the answer, or even why the question is relevant, but read on.

Headings with a shaded square next to them relate directly to a question posed in my questionnaire. You'll find a wealth of information, tips and ideas. You'll become more aware of what you can do yourself to bolster your physical and emotional health, and more aware also of how you can be an informed patient. Next time you go to see your GP you'll be empowered to play a part in your own health care.

My wish is that this book will get you oriented into a way of living and thinking that will make you healthier, happier, and less likely to succumb to illness. But this is also a reference book that I hope you will revisit frequently. It takes time for new ideas to be absorbed, and, often, fresh experiences are needed to put things into context and act as the catalysts of change – which is the goal where ultimate health is concerned.

Deborah McManners

PART 1

Finding a Balance

CHAPTER 1

The McManners Method

As a doctor I have always worked hard to give my patients the most thorough diagnosis and appropriate treatment. But very early in my career I had to accept that the conventional medical training I had received would not fully equip me to do this.

Doctors, as a profession, generally fail to pay enough attention to holistic health – the art of treating the individual as a whole, and not just as a set of symptoms. The benefits of nutrition and exercise are known, but often too poorly communicated to those in our care. Complementary medicine is often patchily understood, neglected or dismissed.

I come from a fairly bohemian family, and was brought up on common-sense 'naturopathic' principles for healthy living. So as a medical student, I saw no reason to accept – as so many doctors have tended to do – that patients on lower incomes and with relatively poor levels of education would die ten years or so before their more affluent and better educated peers.

What had inspired me to become a doctor was a strong urge to help people help themselves. Of course, I knew that it was no longer possible for all doctors to get to know their patients' underlying problems the way that traditional family doctors did, by visiting their homes and seeing for themselves how they were living. But such things as a person's diet, the way they heat their home, the pets they keep, their general happiness – all factors with a huge bearing on our health – can and should be taken into account before a prescription is issued. And, although I pursued an orthodox medical career, my desire to enable people to take control of their own health never left me.

When I became a general practitioner I was frequently surprised at the fact that my patients would hand over a description of their symptoms, then leave me to it – as if their health were my problem, not theirs! What I wanted and tried to give each one was a little insight into the simple things they could do at home to improve their health. This eventually became so important to me that I spent further years training as a naturopath, while also holding down my GP's job and raising my two young sons, William and Joseph.

We have holiday snapshots that show me, fully dressed on the beach, with my head buried in a book. It was a real slog, but the positive feedback I got from my patients more than buoyed me up. And, although it seems like commonsense to me to treat patients naturopathically – ensuring they have the best of what both orthodox and complementary medicine can offer – I was the first female medical doctor in the UK to become a registered naturopath. Although naturopathy is widespread in the US, Australasia and Europe, it remains a young practice in the UK. In fact, there are only a few hundred of us registered with the General Council and Register of Naturopaths, the body that ensures the highest standard of training and regulation in the field.

I was encouraged to write this book, and share the experience I've amassed over the years, by patients at my thriving medical and naturopathic clinics. So here it is! In it, I hope to give you the insight to understand your body and improve your everyday wellbeing and self-esteem.

Total health

I am going to talk you through total health, by which I do not simply mean 'not being ill'. The founding charter of the World Health Organization describes health as 'a state of complete physical, mental and social wellbeing'. For some reason this message has been overlooked or forgotten by many medics. But what it really means, and what I strongly believe, is that the whole of your life should be taken into account when assessing your health – not just your physical or biological health, but also the spiritual, emotional and mental aspects of your life. So my goal is to help you achieve a state of *total* wellbeing.

You may think that all these parts of your life are already in order. But when asked, 'How healthy are you?' most people may say, 'I'm good . . . but I had a cold last month,' or 'Fine, apart from the odd bit of eczema.' Our health is hard for us to define. So, instead of trying to evaluate it, try asking yourself: 'How do I feel when I wake up in the morning?'

Think about how you felt as a child. You probably leapt out of bed, full of energy and looking forward to the day ahead. How long has it been since you felt anywhere near that way – bright-eyed, thoroughly rested and raring to go?

If you've forgotten that feeling, and wake up instead to listlessness, resignation or fatigue, this book is for you. You may have no idea why you feel like this, or what you can do about it. Or you may have tried everything you can think of to solve the problem. A lot of my patients have been up and down London's Harley Street, paying for one expensive test after another, and shelling out for treatments and supplements that never seem to have any long-term effect. Being health conscious can be a very expensive habit! But being healthy (and note the difference, because health-conscious people are not always as healthy as they want to be) can be very simple, and very inexpensive. I believe that with the right approach, anyone can improve and regain his or her vitality.

The following cases are typical of patients I have treated.

- Sue, who had suffered from chronic sinusitis, eczema and constipation for over four years. Her GP had worked through conventional treatments, but with no long-term relief. Now, sadly, she was just another patient number on his records system, still saddled with her problems.

- Jane, who at just 26 was physically exhausted and mentally depleted by her high-flying career. She had reached an impasse and, despite her tender age, believed herself to be 'too old' to make changes to her professional life.

- Charles, who had suddenly become one of the apathetic and constantly tired people he had always despised. His GP could find nothing wrong with him, and Charles was beginning to wonder if it was all in his mind.

- Simon, who developed the embarrassing and debilitating 'old man's disease' prostatitis when he was just 32, at the height of an exciting career in the media.

These four people had completely different health concerns. But like all my patients, all four shared one underlying problem: they lacked balance in their lives. This kind of balance is the key to any individual's health, and it's a concept I want you to understand when thinking about your own state of health.

Balance means having time to yourself as well as time for your work, family and friends. It means making room in your life for things you want to do and not putting them off. To be balanced, you have to give yourself time to eat properly, sleep well and be active, while also making sure that you devote the right amount of time and attention to both your home and work lives.

Most of the time we can tell when we lack balance in our lives, but sometimes we're too stressed or too busy to recognise certain imbalances. I want to help you recognise these.

You have probably heard of 'vital energy' as the central element in producing and maintaining good health. In traditional Chinese medicine it is called Qi (pronounced 'chee'). When Qi is imbalanced or its flow is blocked, health can suffer; acupuncture, herbalism and other techniques can unblock the flow, bring balance back and restore health. Ayurvedic doctors, who practise a form of medicine originating in India five millennia ago, also base their work on balance, harmonising the different elements that contribute to each person's wellbeing. They too rely on the principle that any disorder can be prevented if balance is maintained, not just in the body, but in the mind and spirit as well.

Homeopathy is another system of medicine based on balance – specifically, on the idea that 'like cures like'. The patient's essential physical and emotional make-up are assessed along with their symptoms; then, minute doses of the very substances that would ordinarily trigger those symptoms are prescribed in order to stimulate the body's ability to heal itself and restore its natural balance.

My view of the body's vital energy is that it is constantly fluctuating. Its ebbs and flows are influenced by a multitude of factors, but it must be balanced to maintain health. When this equilibrium is lost we become ill: the symptoms can be a sign that your body is struggling to re-establish the balance it has lost.

My aim in this book is not just to show you how to restore this vital balance, but to help you to strengthen it and build up your reserves to prevent ill health from taking hold. Total health is about looking ahead and building for a healthy future – retaining as well as regaining vitality. We hear a lot these days about demographic change and how people are living so much longer than ever before. But where are all these very elderly people we read about?

Quite a few of them are languishing in long-term care in nursing homes, rather than fulfilling the role of active members of our communities. The lives of people in this situation are sadly restricted: they've lost their mobility and independence and may suffer degenerative disorders such as Alzheimer's. They have longevity, but little freedom and a poor quality of life – and who wants that? As I write this I have just been playing cards with a friend – a 96-year-old great-grandmother who has just told me how to make wonderful pumpkin and cinnamon jam. She's waiting for the arrival of another baby in her family, and has certainly not lost her zest for life. That is how I would like to be at 96. My own grandmother was very similar and still knew how to party at that age! To me, total health is about achieving both longevity *and* quality of life.

The McManners Method

Thanks to both my upbringing and my training as a naturopath, I've developed a philosophy of health and healing quite different from a purely conventional doctor's. The term naturopathy means 'healing through nature', and that is its essence: it's based on Hippocrates's *vis medicatrix naturae*, a principle which holds that all living things have an innate power to heal themselves. So I may use conventional treatments, but I also use therapies that involve simple, natural elements such as good nutrition, sunlight or water, to help enhance your powers of self-healing.

LET THE FORCE BE WITH YOU

Essentially we are built to survive, and we need to harness and assist this vital force or healing energy to enable our bodies to have the best chance of good health and vitality. It is also essential to address and as far as possible remove what are known as 'obstacles of cure' – obvious examples include an excess of alcohol or too many late nights.

As both a naturopath and conventional doctor, my practice is guided by seven basic beliefs:

1. Do no harm.

2. Nature has healing powers.

3. Identify and treat the cause of illness, not just the symptoms.

4. Treat the whole person, and treat them as an individual.

5. The physician is a teacher.

6. Prevention is the best cure.

7. Establish and maintain health and wellness.

There are acute situations where conventional treatment must be used immediately. And where a problem is chronic, and has troubled the sufferer for a long time, it is equally important to evaluate the condition conventionally – but a naturopathic approach can make a great difference to the management of the complaint.

So although a conventional doctor might consider the job done once you have recovered from your initial symptoms, my approach would be to work with you to treat the underlying causes of ill health, and also to boost your reserves of energy. This increases the capacity of your mind and body to withstand disturbance and regain equilibrium if your defences are challenged.

This way of combining medical and naturopathic management is a process whereby you learn to become a healthier person overall by improving every aspect of your health. My patients learn to understand and manage their own conditions, with help and guidance from me. Together our ultimate goal is to prevent future illness and establish long-lasting health and wellness.

The triangle of health

Your health and wellbeing are governed by three elements in constant flux: your biochemistry, your physical state and your psychology. Together they form the three corners of a triangle that represents your total health.

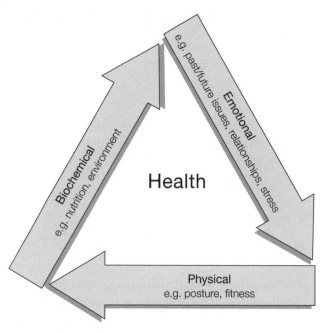

Naturopaths use the triangle of health to represent your *total* health

This triangle of elements governs my approach to health and healing, guiding my diagnosis and treatment. When I teach patients how to reach and maintain total health, I use the triangle to convey how total health means building and maintaining reserves of biochemical, physical and psychological health. You'll find that most of this book follows this three-fold structure.

I'll be talking about each aspect of health – each corner of the triangle – separately, but in reality, they all work together to maintain your overall health. And they are all equally important.

How does it work? Take a common problem like weight gain or an inability to lose weight, for example. To control weight you have to:

- **Watch your diet.** What you eat and when you eat it will affect your body's ability to maintain a steady weight. Eating high-energy junk food and large meals late in the evening, for example, can exacerbate a weight problem. This is all part of your biochemical health.

- **Do enough exercise.** Having more muscle than fat on your body accelerates your metabolism. Exercise is also a way of burning off unwanted fat stores. This is all part of your physical health.

- **Keep stress under control.** When we are under stress, we often don't feel we can take time out for exercise, or are too worn out to get going in the evenings – our workload or anxieties take over. Stress hormones like cortisol then cause us to store fat as an energy supply. Stress is also behind a lot of comfort eating. How you cope with stress is part of your psychological health.

This is a very clear and straightforward example of the health triangle. Often, however, it's a bit harder to apply this model to your health problem. That is why I treat patients holistically, and encourage them to examine all corners of their own lives for clues about imbalances which may connect in some way to their current state of health.

Let's take a closer look at the three 'corners'.

Biochemical health

This corner causes the most confusion, because it's enormously complex and varied: it covers every chemical and biological process at work in your body, along with the internal and external factors that influence them. Your biochemical health is influenced by everything from the detoxification enzymes at work in your liver to the allergenic particles in the air around you. It also includes your diet and digestion – and nutrition is an important element of this corner.

Physical health

This corner covers the physical aspects of your body: the structural elements of bone, muscle, cartilage and tendon, as well as the health of your heart, lungs and other major organ systems. An active life is the key to health in this corner of the triangle. Other important factors include posture, breathing and ergonomics (how we sit, stand, breathe and use, or misuse, our bodies).

Psychological health

The third corner of the triangle is psychological health, which I sometimes refer to as 'mento-emotional' health because it covers all aspects of your mental and emotional life, including the spiritual. Once again, balance is key. Good psychological health involves a sense of inner equilibrium, but this is often shaken by events – some of which may have happened many years ago. Turning points in your life can have a dramatic impact, and I always ask patients about regrets they may have put behind them after decisions, for example about which degree course to take, or which career path to follow. A lost opportunity, even if you haven't recognised it as a loss at the time, can really upset the apple cart, leading to nebulous health problems in later life. I remember sitting next to a scientist at a medical conference talking about my son's ambition to be a solo violinist – he too had once had this dream. It is very hard to become a violinist at this level, but, as he said to me, 'It is even harder *not* to be a violinist.'

Often we are on such a treadmill that we don't stop to think about what we really want from life. But it's vitally important that this aspect of well-being is not overlooked. As the poet W.H. Davies so rightly asks: 'What is this life if, full of care, we have no time to stand and stare?'

Where's your weakness?

George, Alison and Caroline all came to me with very typical modern complaints. But when we considered their conditions using the triangle model, we saw that each had a weakness at a different point of it.

George had chronic rhinitis (nasal stuffiness). He relied heavily on antihistamines, yet found he couldn't enjoy his life or give the time he wanted to his volunteer work. A detailed medical history and thorough physical examination revealed a biochemical weakness: it turned out that George had a food intolerance. We were able to overcome this, enabling him to lead a normal, healthy life again.

Alison suffered from chronic headaches and was taking huge amounts of painkillers – but they had little effect. She came to me because she wanted to find a more natural approach to treating the problem. When I looked into her biochemical, psychological and physical health, I found something that her own GP had missed – in fact, something many conventional doctors may never have routinely looked for, given her symptoms. Alison had a curvature of the spine in her lower back. This was interfering with her posture and, in turn, triggering headaches. As well as suggesting ways in which she could build up her physical health reserves, I referred her to an osteopath who helped her strengthen her back and improve her posture. Her headaches cleared.

Caroline had serious irritable bowel syndrome (IBS), a condition that causes abdominal pain, bloating and alternating constipation and diarrhoea. IBS can have a biochemical or physical basis, but it can also be triggered by psychological trauma. And in fact, when Caroline and I discussed her childhood, we uncovered the fact that at 14 she had suddenly lost her 18-year-old brother in a road accident. Her unresolved grief – what is often called 'unfinished business' – had knocked her off balance psychologically. This had affected the rest of her health. Just recognising the problem helped her start to deal with it, and although she needed some professional counselling, her equilibrium was eventually restored – and she wasn't troubled by IBS again.

Putting it all into practice

By examining each of the elements of the triangle, you can build up a definition of your own health that will help you to recognise where and how you need to make changes. If you can achieve this, you can identify your priorities and set realistic health and lifestyle goals. When you use the triangle model, you will often realise you need to reassess your priorities so that no one area of your life is allowed to become unbalanced. It's not always easy . . . but it is always possible.

Take my own life, which is pretty complicated with an awful lot of demands on my time. I have a busy practice and I do a lot of work in the media, but I also want to live in the countryside, have an active life, maintain a healthy lifestyle and, above all, raise a family. I see patients in London and country clinics, maintain a large country house, keep several horses as well as livestock, am active on local conservation and environmental issues, take a lot of exercise, eat well, encourage my sons to develop their musical careers and spend a lot of time with my husband. So how do I do it?

The key is keeping my priorities in focus. Without the firm family foundation that I have built, I would not be so effective in other areas of my life. I arrange my time carefully, draw on the support of my husband and kids, delegate where necessary and try not to bite off more than I can chew. I may not have it all arranged perfectly, but I manage to have a full and fulfilling life. And in fact it's *because* I manage to be true to myself and my priorities that I have the reserves to accomplish all this. *Because* I invest so much time in being with my family, taking exercise, being in the countryside, riding horses, living a healthy lifestyle, getting involved with the local community and so on, I manage to build up my reserves in every corner of the triangle and stay healthy and happy. If I lost sight of this balance and concentrated too much on any one aspect of my life – my career, for instance – then my reserves would drain away and it could all fall apart. I would be doing what I see so many of my patients doing: 'missing the point'.

Time and again I see people who are no longer enjoying life. Men who have been on a career treadmill only to wake up one day and say, 'where did my thirties go?', and who feel they are hurtling towards 50; women in their late thirties who say they're not ready for children 'yet' (even though their partners may be champing at the bit) because they 'don't have time right now'. Unhappiness and misplaced priorities affect our psychological health – often with physical consequences. So now it's your turn to ask yourself the big question. *Are you missing the point? Are you enjoying life?* If everything were to end now, would you feel you'd spent your time well? Are you happy with where you're going and how you're getting there? Are you looking after all three corners of your own personal triangle of health and building reserves of health for the future?

The aim of this book is to help you achieve psychological, biochemical and physical health. The very first step along that road is to learn to judge how close you are to achieving good health in all three areas, where the gaps are, and what you need to do to close them.

CHAPTER 2

Tales from my casebooks

W hen I was a general practitioner working full time within the
National Health Service, the free healthcare system that we have
enjoyed in England since the end of the Second World War, a fair proportion
of my patients clearly felt that good health was something their doctor
should deliver and was in fact wholly responsible for. Over the last 20 years,
advances in medical technology have led people to expect much more from
their doctors, while simultaneously eroding their sense of responsibility for
their own health.

I am very much in favour of healthcare for all according to their need, but
this need seems to increase every year. The founding father of the NHS,
Aneurin Bevan, believed that once healthcare was funded by the state, the
populace would eventually become so healthy that the running costs of the
system would fall. Sadly, he was wrong. When people see the state as the
absolute guardian of their own and their families' health, they relinquish
their sense of responsibility for achieving and maintaining it – and all too
often, their wellbeing goes out the window.

Patients who come to see me are entering into a very different sort of
relationship. As a medical doctor and a naturopath I set great store in my
role as a teacher. Discussion, understanding and a strong sense of teamwork
are a vital part of the process. I always urge my patients to make sure they
learn something during each consultation – not simply attend surgery in

order to be treated. We discuss how they can make changes, and how to put into practice what has been discussed during the consultation.

With my patients, I work hard to develop a high level of 'patient responsibility' – a catchphrase these days, but one that encapsulates that vital notion, a willingness to work towards one's own health. I use the 'art' of medicine here, which I find sits very comfortably alongside scientific medicine, to lessen the chances of ill health, and to improve a person's overall health. I explain the naturopathic triangle of good health, and how the aim is not only to manage the complaint, but also to build nutritional, physical and emotional reserves as part of a lifestyle in which ill health is less likely.

This does not mean that we all have to live like Puritans. It means that with the right information, we can make choices that will improve rather than drain our wellbeing. It's a trade-off between, for example, feeling lousy in the morning, having poor concentration or feeling stiff and heavy – common symptoms of less than optimal health – and the inconvenience of making changes that make us feel better.

Taking action

My approach to good health is *active*, through everyday living. The alternative is *passive*, in which a person accepts sub-optimal health with episodes of ill health from time to time. In time this will lead to a dependency on the medical profession to 'fix' the problems, rather than a determination to make the necessary changes to our lifestyles.

One of the most common things that I see in my patients is general fatigue – that 'tired-all-the-time' feeling. Although it is a doctor's job to exclude underlying illness by listening to and examining their patient, and ordering the appropriate investigations, very often doctors don't find any clear medical reason why a person might feel below par, wake unrefreshed and struggle through the afternoon at work – let alone have the energy to go to the gym. Doctors are seeking organic physical diseases, quite rightly, but if they don't find evidence of one, they will often classify the problem as a functional disorder or psychosomatic illness.

Another good example is irritable bowel syndrome (IBS), which I discussed briefly in Chapter 1. This common and sometimes chronic complaint involves intermittent diarrhoea and constipation, abdominal pain and bloating. IBS can only be diagnosed after all other possible causes of these symptoms (bowel polyps, inflammation or cancer) have been considered and ruled out, but the management of IBS shows how important it is to consider all three points of the health triangle.

There could be a nutritional cause. The sufferer may, for example, have a low tolerance for certain foods, a condition which can only be pinned down through tests or an elimination diet. Or he may have gut dysbiosis – an abundance of unhealthy gut flora, leading to fermentation and gas formation in the intestine.

A physical factor may be to blame. One accountant told me that he was sitting at his desk for up to 16 hours a day, so it's hardly surprising that his bowel habit and intestinal functions were disturbed.

Emotional factors have to be explored as well: what causes a man to spend such long hours at his desk? Is it the urge to succeed or the fear of failure that drives them the most?

Quite often, the first thing people tell me when we have a follow-up consultation is that their energy levels have improved. This is always a very good indication that their bodies are adjusting to naturopathic treatments.

Andrew was a case in point. Referred to me by a urologist colleague of mine, Andrew had chronic prostatitis, an inflammation of the prostate gland that causes significant pain and disability. The complaint can be quite resistant to conventional treatment. More, Andrew could not even sit down during his first consultation. Aside from the painful prostatitis, he had a 20-year-old spinal fusion – surgery to stop two vertebrae rubbing by 'welding' them together. On top of it all, he was suffering from classic IBS, with periodic constipation and abdominal pain. He could no longer drive and hardly went to the opera, which he loved, as he could not sit for long periods. In short, he was a very unhappy man. But a combination of dietary approaches and physical therapy for his back vastly improved all his symptoms. To my delight, he declared after eight weeks that he felt better than he had in 20 years – and he has maintained this improvement long-term.

Beyond 'okay'

As a naturopathic approach aims to improve *overall* health and wellbeing, I aim to give advice that a person can follow to build health reserves. My goal, for the people who come to see me, is to help them go beyond feeling merely 'okay' and being symptom-free to achieving a state of superhealth. They should have physical, emotional and nutritional reserves to draw upon when stressed by some crisis (whether that be flu or an emotional upset). Then the likelihood of their returning to a healthy equilibrium is greater, and they'll manage it far more speedily, too.

In routine medical practice, when a person develops a physical ailment, they will consult with their doctor to gain an understanding of what is wrong and how to overcome the problem. The doctor will then often advise a medication-orientated approach to recovery, and offer helpful advice. During an integrated naturopathic medical consultation, however, we address all the issues – physical as well as emotional – as a matter of course. This may seem incongruous in a routine appointment, but it's clearly a more holistic approach with real advantages for both doctor and patient. Nevertheless, it does require commitment on both sides.

Fiona came to see me about her hay fever. This was her first visit, so I took a full account of her problems and her life in general. When I go through this process with new patients, the huge advantage of following both medical and naturopathic principles is highly evident: no stone is left unturned. And there are patterns that will emerge only when information about the patient's physical symptoms is pieced together with the emotional, well-being and lifestyle factors that emerge during the consultation. I structure the interview in such a way as to understand the patient in the context of their life, their past and the people around them.

Fiona lived in London but her family had moved to Canada. I learned that her sister had recently been diagnosed with bowel polyps. This condition, which may run in families, increases the risk of a person developing cancer. Obviously, as a doctor, I first had to examine her 'presenting complaints', in this case hay fever, but at the same time I was actively looking for issues such as a history of family illnesses, other physical problems, her emotional state and any social issues. During this process, the need for conventional medical investigations like blood samples and specialist tests often becomes apparent, so I referred her for a colonoscopy – an internal investigation of the entire colon.

The examination revealed that she too had bowel polyps, despite being completely free of any symptoms to indicate this might be a possibility.

These were removed and tested for cancer – which happily was not present. Now the risk of her developing a life-threatening tumour is very greatly reduced, as she will have colonoscopies at intervals as advised by her specialist to remove and screen any polyps.

Fiona's case is a good example of the importance of taking a very full history even when someone comes in with a specific complaint. In the event, the polyps were the obvious priority, but we also manage her hay fever very successfully.

Throughout this book I will be encouraging you to take a holistic approach to your own health. This means, as we've seen, considering all possible links to your symptoms and concerns, no matter how tenuous they may appear to be.

PART **2**

Biochemical Health

CHAPTER 3

What are you doing to your body?

Do you eat a healthy diet, but seem unable to shed those excess pounds? Is your hay fever getting worse every summer, but you can't figure out why? Are you cursed with mysterious mid-afternoon slumps when you can hardly keep your eyes open? Since I qualified as a doctor in 1983, I have seen more and more people suffering from weight gain, allergies and fatigue – all conditions very likely to have a biochemical basis.

Remember that biochemical health has to do with all the chemical and biological processes in your body, as well as factors that influence them – particularly diet, digestion and stress. So when patients arrive suffering from symptoms such as the ones above, we'll talk about what they're eating and how they live – filling up on refined carbohydrates and saturated fats, perhaps, or rushing around to meet deadlines and never having a clear desk or that blessed sense of 'empty space'. There's always something we're in a hurry to do, it seems, and to keep up we might find ourselves relying on fast energy boosts such as sweets and chocolate, with little thought for the longer-term effects.

The following chapters will help you evaluate your own biochemical health. But to get the most out of them, you will first need to take out a bit of time to write up a food diary.

This need only be a rough record of what you ate and when over a week. As well as your main meals, you will need to record all drinks, snacks and extras such as oil used in cooking, sugar added to tea, milk poured on cereal and so on. Note whether food is organic, and the degree to which it has been processed (was it tinned or a packaged meal; and if it was an apparently fresh food like a salad, was it pre-washed and packaged?).

Finally, as well as your 'inputs' (what you've had to eat and drink), you need to keep a record of your outputs – the frequency and quality of your urine and stool. If you're grimacing at this prospect, let me reassure you that you're not alone. Most of my patients look horrified when I ask them to start looking at what they have produced in the loo. But the output from your system is an important indicator of how well it is functioning, and we will discuss its implications in Chapter 11.

Anatomy of a food diary

As a doctor, I find food diaries extremely revealing. Not only do they tell me what someone has been eating, but how they tend to eat – and a bit more about what kind of person they are. Do they graze or binge? Do they pick at their food or eat indiscriminately? Are they creatures of habit who stick to the same mealtimes every day? Or do they eat erratically, often skipping meals? Do they think they are healthy eaters? Are they bothered about their diet? Do they eat almost identical meals every day? Or are they truly adventurous, always willing to try something new?

I learn a lot, too, from the way in which this information is recorded. Some patients get so involved with the project that they supply me with reams of neatly typed pages. Others have clearly scribbled their diaries in a hurry. But nearly all become so enthusiastic about the project that, when asked to record five days, they will give me at least seven!

Before we get down to analysing your food diary, let's look at one I kept for a week.

Day 1

Breakfast: unsweetened organic oat porridge with soya milk and an apple

Mid a.m: pumpkin seeds and freshly picked blackberries

Lunch: avocado, toast with olive oil, salad leaves with cucumber, tomatoes, radishes and red onion

Mid p.m: two apples

Dinner: wild venison stew with peas, broccoli and potato.

Day 2

Breakfast: 2 scrambled eggs on wholemeal toast, a glass of banana and strawberry juice

Mid a.m: one apple, hummus on oat cakes

Lunch: Bean salad, olive oil on wholemeal bread with a sun dried tomato, green leaves and onion

Mid p.m: four plums and some yogurt

Dinner: ratatouille with beans and chickpeas.

Day 3

Breakfast: dairy yogurt with oat and millet cereal, dried fruits and a fresh pear

Mid a.m: pumpkin seeds and a banana

Lunch: sardines with organic brown rice salad, tomatoes and cucumber

Mid p.m: berries and an apple

Dinner: wild salmon, beans, broccoli and a large baked potato.

Day 4

Breakfast: organic oat porridge with soya milk and a glass of carrot juice

Mid a.m: two stem ginger balls, goat's milk yogurt and berries

Lunch: organic brown rice, a cold hard-boiled egg, cold ratatouille and an apple

Mid p.m: pumpkin seeds, two plums and some leftover cold porridge

Dinner: shepherd's pie made with organic lamb, carrots, peas and lots of potato mashed with olive oil and braised onions.

Day 5

Breakfast: organic oat porridge with soya milk; fresh apple and berry juice

Mid a.m: hummus, crudités and seeds

Lunch: slab of cold salmon with a dairy yogurt raita, rice and salad

Mid p.m: fresh apple and blackberry juice

Dinner: tuna steak with herbs, swede mashed with cheese and pepper, runner beans.

I also drink good coffee about three times a week, tea about five times a week, filtered or mineral water freely, and a glass of red wine twice a week.

If my diary looks just too perfect or actually daunting, don't let it put you off! As I've said, I grew up in a fairly bohemian family – and even in the 1970s I was taking homemade goats' milk yoghurts and muesli to school in my packed lunches (to the fascination to my classmates). I have always eaten a range of fresh fruit and vegetables and grains, too. But if your own eating habits revolve around less healthy options, such as a lot of fried foods or refined carbohydrates, be aware that I don't expect you to make any drastic changes to your diet overnight. What I am always looking for, instead, is the chance to inspire people to make simple, healthy changes that will remain with them for life. From this point they can slowly build up their nutritional reserves.

Bob was a case in point. A taxi driver, Bob used to take me 300 miles from Kent to Manchester once a week to record for a TV show. Our journey was always punctuated with service station stops, where Bob would tuck into his usual pie and chips, or all-day breakfast. He was already overweight, and heading for the kind of health problems we read so much about; diabetes, heart disease, even cancer are all big risks when you're carrying too much weight. I couldn't sit back and ignore what he was doing to himself – but nor could I expect him to give up the habits of a lifetime overnight. After much chatting about what I do, and what this means in practical terms, he asked my advice and I was able to persuade him to make little changes. I suggested he put a whole plate of green beans or salad on his tray alongside his bacon roll or pork pie, and he found this easy to do. Every fresh vegetable dish he ate was better than none, and would afford him some protection from ill health. And, with luck, it would inspire him to make further healthy changes to his diet and lifestyle.

Kate's food diary showed she always ate the same breakfast (a *pain au chocolat*) and lunch (a tuna and mayo sandwich on white bread). In the afternoon she ate chocolate biscuits. Dinner was predictable, too – chicken featured several times a week in different sauces, rice and pasta were always the white, refined variety. Once a week Kate had a baked potato loaded with butter and cheese, and a rich mayonnaise coleslaw. Keeping to set meals made shopping and cooking easier, something she could tick off her 'to-do' list.

After analysing her food diary and talking to me about changes she should make, Kate began varying her breakfasts so she would sometimes have porridge or sometimes yogurt and fruit, or wholemeal toast with a banana. For lunch she started to make her own soups, or had an avocado salad with wholemeal bread, or sardines on wholemeal toast. For dinner, she started to cook more fish and was surprised at how quick and easy it was. She ordered a surprise box of mixed varieties of fish from an organic supplier, and fully enjoyed the creative challenge of finding ways to prepare and serve the salmon, trout, plaice and mackerel that arrived.

So now you've kept your food diary for a week – congratulations! You may have already been surprised by what you've noted down. Maybe you can notice certain patterns emerging, or you've discovered that, for example, you eat a lot more salty snack food than you thought you did! In the next few chapters, we'll keep coming back to the food diary. I can't stress enough how important it is to be aware of what you're putting into your body. What you eat can have more fundamental effects than you might think.

CHAPTER 4

Healthy eating basics

At medical school I remember spending just one day studying nutrition. I knew then that this was woefully inadequate. Diet plays a huge part in the promotion and prevention of disease. The typical Western diet, for instance, is linked to a number of so-called 'diseases of civilisation', such as late-onset (type 2) diabetes, irritable bowel syndrome (IBS), some cancers and heart disease. These diseases are relatively uncommon in less developed parts of the world, but a number of studies have shown that as populations adopt a more Western diet (as a result of either migration or economic development) the incidence of such problems shoots up – a cautionary reminder that the diet many of us have taken for granted (often for life) may be paving the way for health problems we have the power to prevent.

Eating 'well' means different things to different people. For the gourmet, it may mean fine *foie gras* and a rare vintage. For the rushed mother, it may mean a homemade meal instead of one from a packet. For the office worker, it may mean a sandwich stuffed with chicken mayonnaise and salad from the nearest takeaway. Eating 'well' does not always equate with eating healthily. Go back to the food diary I asked you to keep in the last chapter, and take a good look at what you are usually eating, and think about how well you are really eating.

Now look at the questions on the following pages. Some of them deal with your general 'food IQ', and some with your diet. The remainder of this chapter looks at those questions one by one, aiming to fill any gaps in your basic healthy eating knowledge.

■ Watching what you eat

Would you say that prior to keeping your food diary, you were fully informed and aware of dietary issues and that you kept an eye on what's in the food you eat? Ask yourself the questions below.

- Do you know what constitutes a portion of each of the main food groups (fruit, vegetables, meat, dairy produce, beans, grains/cereals)?

- Over the last week, how many portions of white meat did you eat? How many portions of red meat?

- Over the last week, how many portions of fish did you eat? How many portions of that were oily fish (such as herring, mackerel, sardines, salmon)?

- Over the last week, how many portions of beans and pulses did you eat?

- How many portions of the following did you eat last week (give total for all)? Slices of white bread, processed breakfast cereals, instant potato, sweets, crisps, chocolate, pastries/cake, biscuits, crisps, soft drinks.

- How many units of alcohol did you drink last week?

- How many portions of wholemeal cereals and grains – in wholemeal bread, wholemeal pasta, brown rice, couscous, and cracked wheat or brown or wholemeal cereal/grain products – did you eat last week?

- Over the last week, how many portions of fruit and vegetables did you eat? How many of those portions were green and leafy (think broccoli, not iceberg lettuce!)?

- Over the last week, how many portions of oils and fats (including dairy products) did you eat? How much of that was olive oil/flaxseed oil, dairy fats such as butter and cheese, or animal fats such as hydrogenated fats?

- On average, how much water did you drink per day last week?

How did you rate on the questions in the box above? You may even find, on looking at your food diary, that you're hardly eating any of an entire food group – or that some foods hardly enter your nutritional 'vocabulary' as you just pass them by in the local supermarket. Analysing your food diary gives you invaluable information about yourself, and now we're ready to fill in any gaps in your knowledge by looking at healthy eating in more depth.

What's really healthy?

These days, diet and nutrition get lashings of media attention – so much so, that most of my patients feel they know a great deal about nutrition, and are convinced they're eating healthily. But a closer look often reveals that their eating habits and assumptions about what's normal in terms of weight and body shape need revising.

Justine came to me with what she thought was a weight problem. In fact, when I showed her how to work out her body mass index (her weight to height ratio – see page 192), she realised that she wasn't really overweight at all. In fact, she was quite well down in the 'normal' band, which she was pleased about. But there were serious gaps in her diet. She addressed these, and at the same time learned to separate activities – for example, not eating when watching TV – so she could pay attention to and enjoy her meals.

Marcus was convinced he was eating healthily because he had cereal for breakfast every day. Like so many people, he had swallowed the food manu-facturers' claims that their products form part of a healthy diet. Yes, it's true that grains are crucial to good health . . . but not when they're smothered in sugar and salt!

Sophie told me, 'I hardly ever drink.' But when I asked her for the details, it turned out she was consuming a whole bottle of wine twice a week on girls' nights out. She wasn't drinking on the other days – but without even realising it, she had fallen into the dangerous trap of binge drinking.

No matter how much you think you know about healthy eating, I urge you to keep reading . . . if only to confirm that you really are as knowledge-able as you thought you were!

Back to basics: food groups

Whenever you are evaluating your diet or considering changes to it, it is important to ensure that the essential food groups are all represented. Let's take a look at them. You may feel you learned it all a million years ago at school, but new research has unveiled novel substances in what we eat, as well as shedding light on new features in the old faithfuls.

Proteins   Proteins provide a range of essential amino acids, which are used by the body to ensure healthy growth, metabolism and hormonal functions.

First-class protein sources – meat, fish, eggs and dairy produce – provide the full range of essential amino acids for growth and repair

Second-class protein sources – pulses (chickpeas, lentils and beans), grains (couscous, wheat and rice), and nuts – each provide only some of the essential amino acids and will nearly always need to be eaten in combination (usually a grain with a pulse or nuts) if they are to supply all the essential amino acids you get from a portion of fish or meat (one exception, worth noting if you're a vegetarian, is quinoa, a seed – eaten like grain – that provides the full range of amino acids). But this is not usually too much of a problem. Obvious examples include hummus (made with chickpeas) on wholegrain bread, or a bean stew served with brown rice.

In fact, you only really need to eat regular first-class protein sources if you are in particular need of a rich supply of amino acids – for example, if you are recovering from an illness, or are pregnant or breastfeeding. Regularly adding second-class sources to your diet will get you into the habit of avoiding the saturated fat in meat and cheese, as well as boosting your fibre intake. It's also a good way to learn about different ways of cooking and enjoying food. If you are thinking of becoming a vegetarian, this will be a good introduction – and it will help you avoid the most common pitfall, which is to carry on eating the same foods as before but without the meat! Meals like this will not provide a balanced diet for an adult, and are certainly not sufficient for children and teenagers who require a balanced supply of all nutrients for growth and development. (I see quite a few patients trying to apply their diet to a child, and this is causing a lot of anxiety to health professionals, who call it 'muesli malnutrition'. A high-fibre diet may suit a 33-year-old mum, but if she feeds it to her baby or young child, nasty 'toddler's diarrhoea' may be the result. So let them have seeds and grains, but other foods too!)

In the West we tend to eat far more protein than we need, and in the long term this can lead to problems such as kidney stones and gout. So the main message is to include in your diet what I call the vegetarian protein foods – pulses (beans, lentils, and some soya products), couscous and quinoa – and experiment with them, really getting to enjoy them and make them part of your way of life. After all, on top of all the excellent vegetarian and vegan recipes that have evolved in the West, Latin Americans and Asians have relied on them for centuries. Tapping into their cuisines can be a great voyage of discovery.

Fats and oils   As I have just mentioned, limiting your consumption of meat will help you to cut down on your saturated fat intake. But most of my patients have already got the 'fat is bad' message. For many of them, meat tends to be a rare treat, and olive oil has taken the place of butter. This is great, but the 'fat is bad' dictum seems to have left other, equally vital health messages such as 'eat more fibre'; 'don't skip meals'; and 'monotonous diets are boring too' on the sidelines. Sugar and salt are also big demons. This lopsided view of healthy eating means many of my patients think that skipping lunch every day and eating a low-fat pasta dish at night is good for them.

But there's another, even more important problem with the fat-is-bad campaign. It can, and does, put many people off eating any type of fat. But there are fats and fats, and you need to be eating an adequate supply of the 'good' ones – the essential fatty acids (EFAs) contained in fish, nuts, seeds and their oils. The healthy eating guidelines in this chapter outline how you can get all the EFAs you need without trying, but if you're unsure of your intake use only cold-pressed oil (such as olive, flaxseed or hemp seed, which contains a good range of EFAs and has a lovely nutty flavour – great for salads). Always store oils in a cool, dark place.

Fruit and vegetables   Fruit and vegetables provide fibre, water, micronutrients, vitamins and minerals, and valuable cancer-fighting antioxidants (see page 60), as well as other 'nutraceuticals'. Aim for a variety, and don't imagine everything has to be superfresh, local and expensive. At an army function I attended many years ago, the commanding officer sent back the entire gathering's main course – because it was accompanied by a root vegetable dish. 'This is not "officers' food"!' he said. Why not? Root vegetables may be cheap, but they are an extremely valuable ingredient in a healthy diet. Frozen organic vegetables are also worth exploring if you're short of time for shopping and need easy access to a good range of produce. They're generally frozen within a couple of hours of picking and are a lovely bright colour – a sure sign of freshness. Nor do they 'go off' at the bottom of the vegetable drawer, so they'll be readily available however busy you are.

RAINBOW ON YOUR PLATE: NUTRACEUTICALS

Nutraceuticals – chemicals found in plant sources, notably colourful fruit and vegetables – are emerging as invaluable aids to overall health. The plant chemicals that scientists are getting most excited about are:

- **Flavonoids**. These have anti-cancer actions and are famously found in green tea. (I recommend patients drink this, but, if, like me, you find it makes you feel nauseous, keep it very weak.)

- **Lutein**. This is found in colourful fruit and vegetables and is especially good for the eyes, fighting age-related macular degeneration (a condition affecting the retina which leads to a loss of vision in the centre of your visual field).

- **Lycopene.** This substance helps combat prostate disease and is found in tomatoes cooked with olive oil. One teaspoon of ketchup contains about 1mg of lycopene, while two cooked tomatoes will provide about 10mg – a good daily amount.

Nutraceuticals work as antioxidants, mopping up the free radicals – the by-products of burning (whether from barbecueing food, burning fuel, or even using up energy within a cell) that can trigger many degenerative diseases. Nutraceuticals are thought to influence the cascade of reactions that lead to cancerous or degenerative changes. But, as with any new field in science, where there are perceived benefits, there may also be risks that we do not yet understand. For this reason, ideal doses of supplements of these plant chemicals have not yet been identified. So, erring on the side of caution, I am keener to encourage a good, healthy diet with plenty of brightly coloured fruit and veg than to direct patients towards supplements, unless there are evidence-based reasons to do so. Research in this area is very exciting and is likely to lead to benefits in health and the advice doctors can give.

Carbohydrates High-protein, low-carbohydrate diets are the mantra of the moment. Forget them. I am a firm believer in carbs, which I feel have been unfairly demonised as weight-loss saboteurs. Yes, you should be avoiding processed carbohydrates such as white pasta, cakes, bread and so on, as they're packed with hidden sugars and 'bad' saturated fats. But you should still be eating plenty of complex carbohydrates – and the greater the variety, the better. Mediterranean and Middle Eastern styles of cooking are great ways of getting used to eating more pulses and pasta alternatives such as cracked wheat or couscous. When eating rice, pasta and bread, try to stick to wholegrain versions as much as possible – the less processed, the better. Have baked or boiled potatoes periodically, and experiment with acorn squash and its relatives, which are great mashed or in soups. Beans are valuable carbs and also a great source of isoflavone phytoestrogens, which may have a range of health benefits (see below).

EAT YOUR BEANS: PHYTOESTROGENS

Most people have heard by now that women in Japan have a very low incidence of breast cancer and menopausal symptoms such as hot flushes, while we in the West have much higher levels. It is no coincidence that the Japanese also eat the most isoflavone phytoestrogens, the oestrogen-like derivatives that are most abundant in soya beans. High levels are also found in chickpeas, flageolet beans and lentils. These substances may also contribute to a healthy heart, prostate and breasts. We in the West eat lamentably low levels of pulses and soya products, so it's advisable to up your intake of pulses, beans, lentils, hummous and soy products.

Please don't go overboard here, though. I don't encourage high-dose supplements or an overindulgence in soya products. Phytoestrogens are a relatively young discovery and there is still more to learn about them. As I repeat throughout this book: 'All things in moderation, nothing in excess.'

Fibre   A healthy diet should be fibre-rich. But just like fats, fibre now has a distorted image in the popular imagination. Its roots lie back in the 1970s and 1980s, when we were being advised to eat wheat bran, particularly in cereals, as a quick-fix alternative to more natural ways of adding bulk. Unfortunately, wheat bran contains phytates, which can be moderately nasty on a couple of counts. First off, they inhibit iron absorption – and many people (particularly menstruating women) are already getting too little iron. Bran can also trigger reactions such as abdominal bloating and wind (see page 133) in a small but significant minority of people. So bulking up on loads of bran to keep our bowels healthy isn't really the answer. We need to examine fibre a little more closely.

There are two fibre 'families' – insoluble and soluble. Bran is an insoluble fibre – the type that has a spongelike effect in the gut, soaking up water and swelling to add bulk. Celery and carrots are also rich in it. Soluble fibre (for example in oats) is rather different: it dissolves in the gut to form a kind of gel. It's valuable because it slows the release of glucose into the bloodstream, and has also been shown to reduce cholesterol levels in the blood. Luckily, if you simply follow the carbohydrate guidelines above, you'll have no difficulty in meeting your soluble and insoluble fibre requirements. Wholegrains such as oats, rye and barley, fruits, vegetables and pulses (kidney beans, for instance) have a lot of soluble fibre, and sensible amounts of wholewheat products and fibrous veg will provide the necessary bulk.

◼ What's a portion?

Most of my patients admit to being confused about the size of a portion. If you are too, the following is a good guide:

- **Grains and cereals**: a cupful of cooked rice, oats or millet (or half a cup uncooked), or a thick slice of wholegrain bread. Aim for two portions daily.

- **Beans and pulses**: a cupful (cooked). Aim for one portion at least three times a week.

- **Fruit**: one apple, orange, kiwi, mango, papaya or banana; or two small plums or a cupful of berries. The important thing here is to make sure you vary the fruit you eat. Don't always have the same things. Your daily fruit and vegetable intake should be at least five portions a day.

- **Vegetables**: have four or five cupfuls daily of a variety of vegetables such as peas, runner beans, cauliflower, carrots, tomatoes, broccoli, spinach or kale. Again, aim for a good variety over your week. Count a salad or a stir-fry (with the minimum of oil and a couple of tablespoons of water or veg stock to steam it, so it's really a 'steam-fry') as one portion.

- **Meat and fish**: red meat (lean lamb, beef or pork) – one steak every week or two; white or wild meat (pheasant, turkey, venison, guinea fowl and so on) – 4 to 6oz (120 to 180g) once a week; fish – one trout, one mackerel, a wild salmon steak or a tin of sardines at least three times a week.

- **Dairy**: half a glass of semi-skimmed milk, or 2oz (60g) cheese daily.

- **Eggs** are another valuable source of protein and minerals, and some varieties are rich in omega-3 fatty acids – one, once or twice a week. (The omega-3 content in this kind of egg is determined by the feed the birds are given. This information is often included on the eggbox label.)

- **Fats and oils**: 1 tablespoon of olive or flax oil, or up to ½oz (15g) butter daily. I favour oils, but organic unsalted butter can be part of a good diet.

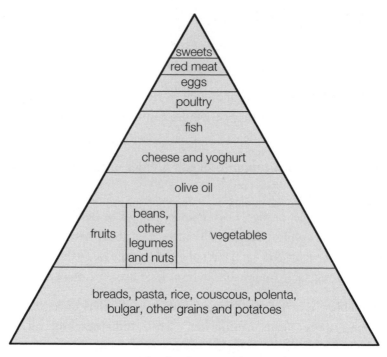

The food pyramid

The portion information above is a handy outline; now let's take a closer look. You may be familiar with the official food pyramid, which outlines the correct proportions of each food group that you should be eating. Take a glance at it (above) and compare it with your answers to the questions on page 28. How do they match up? People in the West typically fall short in the areas of fruit, vegetables, grains and pulses, particularly since in the latter category most of the starchy foods we eat are highly processed and lacking in fibre and micronutrients (see pages 55–6).

■ How many portions of meat?

Your upper limit for meat should be one portion of red meat a week and no more than two portions of chicken a week. In fact I rarely, if ever, tell patients to eat chicken. Despite its reputation for being a healthy low-fat meat (its popularity soared after it was recommended by the Royal College of Physicians and the British Cardiac Society in 1976, and is now our main source of meat in the UK), most is highly processed, intensively reared and pumped full of fat to make it juicy and tender. A wild chicken is a much tougher, highly muscled bird (as I discovered when my sons decided to cook one of our cockerels, which had died of old age – it had huge, muscular legs). If I am recommending low-fat meat, I tend to mean organically reared poultry or wild meats such as guinea fowl, venison and wild boar. Some rare breed pigs (especially woodland reared), from specialist suppliers, are also far lower in fat.

Although meat is an excellent source of iron and amino acids, you must always remember that the saturated fat it contains is a major contributor to heart disease.

HOW FATTY IS IT?

There's ten times more healthy polyunsaturated fat in wild meat than in reared meat, due to the animals' diet and conditions of growth.

I feel that children, however, do need red meat at least once or twice a week, and that vegetarian options must be chosen with great care to ensure an adequate supply of micronutrients. I strongly urge anyone considering a vegetarian diet – especially for their children – to seek expert advice. (See the resources section on page 291.)

■ How many portions of fish?

Ideally you should be aiming to eat around three portions of fish per week – and as much as possible of that should be oily. That would be a small tin of sardines or herring, a wild or organically farmed salmon steak or a mackerel or trout fillet. Oily fish are a good source of protein and low in saturated fat, but high in omega-3 essential fatty acids (EFAs). These are types of fat that your body cannot make for itself and needs for skin and tissue health, wound healing, regulating allergic response and nervous system and cardio-vascular health. If you're eating less than three portions of oily fish per week you could be deficient in omega-3s.

Note, however, that pregnant women are advised to avoid eating more than one portion of tuna, shark, marlin or swordfish a week. These fish can contain mercury and there is some concern that this could accumulate and be potentially harmful to the unborn baby. However, at the moment this guideline only applies to pregnant women, and there is thought to be no significant risk to other adults.

◼ How many portions of beans and pulses?

You've seen that I am a fan of beans. And that's not surprising, given the good they contain: protein, low levels of saturated fat, high levels of beneficial fibre and isoflavones (see pages 33–4) to boot. Ideally, you should be getting a proportion of your protein from beans and pulses. If you eat less than three portions a week, you're not getting enough.

Even though I've mentioned how versatile they are, you may already be groaning at the thought of adding lentils, chickpeas and dried beans to your weekly shop. And I am only too aware that many of my patients stock up on these foods with good intentions – then never bring themselves to open the packets, which remain at the back of their larder out of sight and out of mind. I agree it's daunting to add new foods to your diet. But homemade hummus (using tinned chickpeas for speed, and whizzed up in a blender with olive oil and plenty of garlic until it reaches the right consistency) is an easy dish to start with, as most of us are already familiar with it. And it's well worth making, as a lot of shop-bought hummus is too salty. Try to broaden your range of pulses, though. Throw drained, cooked (or canned) chickpeas, lentils or haricot beans into salads, soups and stews. An easy and delicious supper is to gently cook onions, peppers and tomatoes in a large sauté pan until soft, then add a drained can or cup of haricot or cannellini beans and serve with couscous and perhaps a piece of fish.

◼ How many sugary starchy foods?

Among all the hype and debate about low-fat diets, a problem that's at least as serious is often overlooked. And that is the massive overabundance of simple carbohydrates, such as refined sugar, bread and pasta, in the Western diet. As I've said, I'm a champion of carbohydrates and they are an essential part of your diet; in fact, they should make up around 70 per cent of it, ideally. The crucial issue is, what type of carbohydrate?

When we all embraced Audrey Eyton's high-fibre 'F-plan' regime in the early 1980s, the idea was that we would start to introduce more complex carbs into our diets – wholegrain cereals, wholemeal bread and pasta, and brown rice. Somehow, the message got muddled and now a lot of my patients are labouring under the false impression that their lunchtime baguette sandwich and white spaghetti supper are fulfilling their nutritional requirements. The problem is that white bread and pasta score high on the 'glycaemic index', which measures how fast a food is transformed into blood glucose. And as such, they can cause a surge in blood sugar levels.

If you eat a lot of these foods, as well as sugary cereals, sweets, chocolates, cakes, biscuits and soft drinks, you'll far exceed your blood sugar requirements. You can become exhausted by energy surges and slumps, and the excess glucose in the blood tends to be converted into fat and stored, or can just ferment in your gut (see 'Dysbiosis' below). Habitual consumption of these simple carbs has been linked to a range of modern plagues, such as diabetes, obesity and gut disorders. It is particularly alarming that children in the West are now developing the kind of diabetes (mature onset or type 2) that doctors have always associated with older, overweight patients.

Your food diary should show that you eat hardly anything from this category, and ideally nothing from it at all. But realistically – and in the non-puritanical spirit I favour – just aim to keep your intake down to no more than two or three of these foods a week.

■ How much alcohol?

A unit of alcohol equals, briefly, one glass of wine, half a pint of beer or one shot of spirits. But there's more to it than that.

Do you know how tiny an alcoholic unit really is? I mention this because, these days, most of us own very large wine glasses at home. And when you are out in a bar, pub or restaurant, wine sold by the glass often comes in a choice of two sizes – 175ml or 250ml. In fact, an alcoholic unit of wine is the type of mini wine glass you would have drunk from 30 years ago, or may still get given at the school cheese and wine evening! Next time you have a glass of wine at home, measure it out first. Your unit is 125ml of a 9 per cent 'abv'

Brain activity – too much alcohol is bad for your brain, and scans of the brains of young alcoholics show extensive damage. In fact the brain of a 30-year-old alcoholic looks like the brain of a 50-year-old because alcohol ages it so badly.

PMS – women who drink are more prone to premenstrual mood swings and cravings.

Breast cancer – according to several studies, you've got a higher risk of breast cancer if you drink. One Harvard study found that your risk goes up by about 50 per cent on two drinks a day.

Liver – the damage alcohol does to your liver can increase your risk of potentially fatal cirrhosis, alcoholic hepatitis and liver cancer.

Pancreas – alcohol damages this gland that sits near the stomach. It may cause painful inflammation and increase the risk of pancreatic cancer, which has a poor survival rate.

Osteoporosis – people with excessive alcohol consumption may have bones that look like those of people 40 years older.

Heart – if you already have heart disease, drinking will make your symptoms worse.

Anxiety – you're more likely to have a panic attack within six to twelve hours of drinking, according to some research, and should avoid alcohol completely if it makes you anxious.

Headaches – red wine in particular is a well-known headache and migraine trigger, due to its high content of the chemical tyramine and the fact that alcohol dehydrates.

Heartburn – the irritant effects of alcohol can cause a burning sensation in the middle of the chest, erosion of the stomach lining (gastritis) and a greater likelihood of stomach or duodenal ulcers.

Kidneys – alcohol is a diuretic and excessive drinking can lead to kidney problems.

Blood pressure – there's overwhelming research to prove that alcohol raises blood pressure. And, the more you drink, the higher it goes.

Sex – alcohol increases the risk of short and long term impotence.

Alcohol in pregnancy – I tell patients to avoid alcohol completely when they are either pregnant or trying to get pregnant. Alcohol increases your risk of miscarriage and in extreme cases causes Foetal Alcohol Syndrome which can lead to low birth rate, failure to thrive, cleft palate, heart defects, sleep problems, low IQ and shortness of stature.

What's your poison? How alcohol affects us

(alcohol by volume) wine. And that's something else you should be checking. Most of the wines we drink have a much higher alcoholic content – 11 up to 14 per cent abv. If you've bought this kind of wine, the same size measure (125ml) is the equivalent of one and a half units – so don't have more than two glasses. If your glass is larger, but still what pubs term 'small' (holding 175ml), you will be drinking the equivalent of two units in one glass. If you're a beer or lager drinker, one unit is just half a pint. For spirits, stick to the size of the measure you get in a pub – this is the correct unit measure.

Until recently, government guidelines recommended that women drank no more than 14 units of alcohol a week, while men could drink up to 21 units. Now the figures have been changed and women can have two to three units a day, and men three to four. It looks as if our allowance has gone up. But consistently drinking up to your daily limit is not recommended, and I tell my patients to stick to the 14/21 maximum over a week. The idea is that, even if you drink only once in a blue moon, you should stick to your daily maximum. Women's safe levels are lower than men's because we are physiologically more vulnerable to the effects of alcohol.

Although you won't be doing your health any long-term damage unless you're binge drinking regularly (a binge is officially six units, or about a bottle of wine), having all your units in one go is dangerous and increases your risk of suffering an accident. You're also likely to suffer from the short-term effects of alcoholic poisoning, which will affect the way you feel over the next day or two.

Alcohol problems cost the UK government £3 billion a year, and cause 33,000 deaths – the majority from accidents, alcohol-related liver disease, hepatitis and cirrhosis, and the many cancers which alcohol promotes.

■ How many portions of cereal/grain-based foods?

This figure should be high. Ideally, you'll have eaten six to seven portions of cereal/grain-based foods over the last week, since this food group should be making up a big proportion of your diet to supply the complex carbohydrates and fibre you need. If you've eaten fewer than two portions – and remember, the refined or supersugary stuff like white bread and heavily sweetened cereals don't count – then you're not eating enough. And as a result, you are putting yourself at risk of diseases linked to low-fibre consumption, such as irritable bowel syndrome, bowel cancer and diverticular disease (a condition where the large bowel develops pouches along its length, which can become inflamed and painful and at worst may rupture).

■ How many portions of fruit and vegetables?

Recommendations for fruit and veg intake vary from country to country. The US follows an eight-a-day rule. In Britain it's just five a day, because the government, recognising how poor we were at eating fresh food, could not imagine us finding the time or inclination to eat more than that. Fruit and vegetables are excellent sources of complex carbohydrates, fibre, vitamins and minerals. Leafy green vegetables such as broccoli in particular are rich in fibre and antioxidants – substances that help protect you against cancer, ageing and degenerative diseases.

EIGHT WAYS TO UP YOUR INTAKE OF FRUIT AND VEG

1. Juice. This is such an easy way to get a quick fruit or vegetable fix. Home juicing is best, but if you buy packaged juices, avoid the ones that have had the 'bits' removed, and go for those with the shortest life-spans as they will have been subjected to the least amount of processing. Don't just stick to orange juice, either. These days, there's no excuse as the choice is huge. Try berry juices, vegetable juices and so on. I am always particularly keen to encourage my patients to have a glass of vegetable juice daily.

1. Enjoy 'Swiss muesli'. By this I don't mean the dried cereal and fruit (often with alarming amounts of added sugar) you get in a packet. I was brought up on the old-fashioned Bircher-Benner type muesli that my mother made at home. It's fresh, chopped fruit mixed with live (bio) yogurt, seeds, nuts and grains like oats. (Soak the dry ingredients to make them easier on the teeth.)

3. Snack through the day on a variety of fresh fruits. Focus on the variety – it's too easy to simply sling a banana in your briefcase every day as

---

you head out the door. Try apples, pears, berries, kiwi fruit, satsumas and soft fruit in season.

4. Be inventive with raw vegetables. Make a habit of adding salad leaves, with onion, cucumber, watercress and tomatoes, to lunchtime sandwiches.

5. Cook fruit puddings. Although the cooking makes the fruit slightly less nutritious, a homemade apple and blackberry crumble (with oats and maybe ground nuts in the topping) still has a lot going for it. It's one of my real favourites and always makes me think of home (stew the fruit in a pan first with a lid and very little water – try not to add sugar).

6. Make your own soups. Carrot soup, tomato soup and spinach soup are so easy to make if you have a blender, and you can freeze batches of it too. If you don't think you will get round to this, start with cartons of fresh, low-salt and additive-free soups from the supermarket.

7. Throw fruit into stews and curries. Try fresh apricots in a tagine, or lychees in a curry. Dried fruits also count towards your fruit quota, but check the label to make sure they are unsulphured. Sulphur dioxide is a preservative, and unsulphured dried apricots and cherries are very dark, while the sulphured ones are brightly coloured.

8. Introduce your family to fruit-and-veg starters. Children and adults both like crudités to pick and mix, melon with other fruits, small salads and the like. Chop up carrots, peppers and celery to dip into homemade raita (yogurt with chopped fresh mint), tzatziki (yogurt with cucumber and garlic), or hummus (see page 38).

■ How much fat and oil?

The typical Western diet includes about 40 per cent fat, which is far too high, but as I've already mentioned, the real issue with fat is not only the amount but the type. It's as important to work out how and where your fats and oils came from as it is to know how much of them you ate in total. Fat from animal sources (butter, lard, milk, cheese, meat and so on), margarine or processed vegetable oils, or any oil that's already been used for cooking tends to be bad for you. Fat from sources such as seeds, cold-pressed seed oils, olive oil or fish oils is good for you, mainly because most of these sources supply the EFAs (essential fatty acids) we discussed above.

If more than a third of the portions of fat/oil you ate last week came from butter, margarine, blended vegetable oils and animal fats, you're almost certainly getting too much saturated fat, which boosts your risk of heart disease.

HIDDEN FATS

Beware the fats that lurk in processed foods. These are generally highly undesirable saturated and hydrogenated 'trans' fats. There's a huge amount of evidence that these fats are bad for you but no legislation to get them out of our foods. What can you do? Avoid processed foods!

If none of your fat intake came from seeds, cold-pressed seed oils or fish oils, you're definitely not getting enough EFAs.

■ How much fluid?

In addition to protein, carbohydrates, fats and fibre, there is a fifth major dietary component – water. Use your food diary to estimate your fluid intake, which should ideally be about 2 litres a day. Drink less than this and you put stress on almost every aspect of your internal environment. You'll also increase your chances of problems like constipation and headaches, not to mention tired, dry-looking skin.

But despite a lot of advice to the contrary, water is not the only fluid that counts. Anything that is non-diuretic will keep you hydrated, so drink water by all means, but enjoy weak herbal teas, and fruit and vegetable juices (I dilute mine half and half with water). The risk of dehydration is greater than the supposed risk of over-hydration; but having said that, I do not believe we were ever intended to drink non-stop, and I do worry that some of my patients may be overdoing it by always seeming to have a bottle of water in one hand. Dehydration is a risk when you forget to drink or mistake thirst for hunger (a common mistake), so do have a glass of water if you get a sudden urge to eat something.

HEALTHY EATING BASICS

- Know your food groups

- Check your portions

- Limit refined, processed foods

- Increase fresh and whole foods

- Eat less meat, and more fish

- Have plenty of good-quality complex carbohydrates

- Eat enough EFAs (essential fatty acids) and cut down on saturated fats

- Drink 2 litres of pure water a day

CHAPTER 5

Healthy eating plus

At this point, we've covered all the basics of a healthy diet – proteins, carbohydrates, oils, and fresh fruit and vegetables. And in theory, you could be getting all of these by eating pretty much the same three meals every day. In fact, many of my patients believe themselves to be eating a healthy diet by doing just that! But even though they are getting several portions of, say, 'grains' in a day, they aren't getting any variety. A typical example is pasta. A lot of people fill their grain requirement with this instead of looking around for alternatives such as brown rice, quinoa or couscous.

In the West at least, many people pass entire categories of food by – nuts and seeds (and their oils) and beans and pulses are good examples. And relatively few people today eat foods such as millet, sunflower seeds or flax oil ... yet these are rich sources of important nutrients.

In this chapter I want to help you improve your diet so that it builds up your vital reserves instead of draining them. We'll cover the issue of food quality and try to get to the bottom of the more contentious aspects of nutrition, such as whether, and when, supplements are useful.

Again, look back at your food diary, and now try to answer the questions on the next page. You'll find answers to the questions – and more details – in the rest of the chapter. If it doesn't feel like you're doing very well so far, don't worry. I'll be giving you lots of tips and ideas for improving your diet throughout this section.

■ Gauging the quality of your food

- For each category of the food pyramid (see page 36), how many different foods did you eat? Look back at your food diary to find out.

- Which of the following do you regularly eat? Seeds such as sunflower, pumpkin, sesame and flax; grains such as millet, quinoa, couscous, buckwheat and bulgur wheat; pulses such as lentils, chickpeas and beans.

- How many of your last 10 meals did you make from mainly fresh ingredients?

- How many of your last 10 portions of vegetables did you eat either raw or steamed?

- Do you store your cooking oils in a cool, dark place?

- What proportion of this week's food shopping was organic?

- How many meals (including breakfast) did you skip in the last week? Is there a pattern to the meals you miss?

- How many times in the last week did you eat dinner less than three hours before going to bed?

- Over the last week, how many minutes, on average, did you take to actually eat your lunch?

- Could you have extra nutritional requirements? Are you elderly, pregnant, lactating, on the Pill, menstruating, alcoholic, a smoker, a vegan or vegetarian, or do you have any disorder of the intestinal system? Are you recovering from an illness or injury? Or are you excluding certain foods (such as dairy products) from your diet, without paying attention to the nutrients such as calcium that you may now be lacking?

- Do you have any of the following symptoms?
  - Recurrent mouth ulcers

- Dry, cracked lips or cracking at the corner of the mouth
- Sore tongue
- Red, greasy skin on your face – especially on the sides of your nose
- Rough, sometimes red, pimply skin on your upper arms and thighs
- Scrotal or vulval dermatitis/itch
- Skin conditions such as eczema, dry, rough skin
- Poor hair growth (less than 1 centimetre a month)
- Bloodshot, gritty, sensitive eyes
- Night blindness
- Brittle or split nails
- White spots on your nails
- Pale complexion

Food, glorious food!

Switch on the telly, and you may well find yourself staring at the face of yet another celebrity chef. Your local supermarket's magazine racks are crammed with food and cooking titles, and its aisles are bulging with 'gourmet' this and 'luxury' that. We're food-obsessed; but with what kind of food?

If you aren't already eating a healthy diet, one reason may be that you are afraid you'll have to give up the delectable treats – elaborate designer sandwiches, hand-cooked crisps and huge goblets of wine – to which you've become accustomed. Many of my patients would far rather stick to their present diet, but maybe eat a little less of certain things, and take the odd supplement to make up for all the unhealthy things they eat. As one – a rather overweight man – said to me, 'Can't you just give me something that will do the trick quickly?'

The fact is, healthy eating isn't quite that simple . . . But before you put this book down and give up, let me remind you that I am far from puritanical. My number one principle is – Enjoy Your Food! I do not want you, or any of my patients, to become obsessed with avoiding certain foods or combinations of foods. Apart from making you extremely boring, this kind of obsession can cause a huge amount of stress and anxiety.

The aim of this chapter is not to get you to adopt a 'fad' diet for a couple of weeks and then slip back into your old dietary habits. Nor is it simply to get you to 'tack on' a few foods to an inadequate diet, or learn nutritional quick-fixes. To make any changes lasting, you need to enjoy them.

But with so many different theories around about what we should and shouldn't eat for our health, a lot of people are feeling extremely confused. So what is the ideal diet?

Each of us has his or her own specific biochemistry, so what's ideal for one won't be for another. It's just not possible to come up with a single diet that provides optimum nutrition for everyone. The healthy eating guidelines issued by the government and health agencies are just that – guidelines. They are intended to provide a framework within which to think about your own diet, and it's best to think of them as good advice rather than rules. This chapter works along the same principles, although I have included a few specific diet plans at the end.

■ How varied is your diet?

Use your food diary to see where your diet lacks variety and which food types you're avoiding completely. Then start thinking of ways to explore what's out there.

Do you have the all-too-common cereal/sandwich/pasta habit so many people find themselves stuck in these days? Try steering yourself towards the supermarket aisles you've tended to avoid. Jettison the wheat-based bread and pasta for a few days and substitute brown rice (great with vegetable stir-fries), quinoa (excellent with tomato-based bean stews), bulgur wheat (delicious topped with creamy mushroom sauces made with yogurt), couscous (made for vegetable or organic lamb tagine), rye bread, homemade oat muesli or porridge, and the like.

Be adventurous with the meat you eat – if you've never cooked venison or pheasant, now is the time to experiment. If you imagine you dislike sardines, check out the jars of them from Portugal, which can be true gourmet treats – and add a blast of omega-3 into the bargain. Don't forget pulses: try buying three different kinds of beans – borlotti, flageolet and cannellini, for instance

– and adding them to homemade minestrone. Buy some of the green leafy veg you may have wondered about – bok choy and kale are good lightly steam-fried – and don't stint on fruit. Get a papaya for a delicious breakfast (squeeze half a lime over half the fruit, after scooping out the seeds), or make a salad of kiwi fruit, pears and melon for an after-lunch treat.

■ What was the quality of the food you ate last week?

A fundamental flaw in many official dietary programmes and guidelines is that they fail to recognise that quality is as important as quantity when it comes to food. You can eat a cartload of poor-quality vegetables and not get a huge amount of goodness from them.

Food quality is affected by the way that the food is grown, processed, stored, prepared and cooked. All of these processes can damage or destroy many of the vital nutrients in food, while increasing levels of potentially dangerous contaminants and toxins, such as food additives and agrochemical residues (from fertilisers, pesticides and the like).

We've already covered some issues of food quality in the last chapter. For instance, complex, wholegrain, minimally processed carbohydrates tend to be the highest quality. Wholemeal and brown bread, pasta and rice are definitely better for you than refined, highly processed white bread, pasta or rice. Many of my patients believe they are eating a healthy diet, yet they are not including sources of vegetable protein such as seeds, grains such as millet, quinoa and bulgur or pulses such as lentils and beans.

■ How many of your last 10 meals did you make from mainly fresh ingredients?

If the answer is less than eight – and this includes visits to restaurants and packaged lunches from the supermarket – you're eating too much processed food. The more food is processed, the more vitamins and minerals it loses, the more refined its carbohydrate content becomes, and the more fat, sugar and salt is added. Junk food and pre-prepared meals (such as microwave meals or 'boil-in-the-bag' dishes) may consist of food that has been processed several times, until there's very little goodness left and a lot of dodgy ingredients.

The British government is increasingly concerned about state healthcare costs related to our dependence on these foods. It is now working with the food industry in a move to cut sugar and salt content.

■ How many of your last 10 portions of vegetables did you eat either raw or steamed?

Vegetables are chock-full of health-giving nutrients, but these are easily damaged or destroyed in the cooking process – they can be literally 'done to death'. Any vegetables are better than none, but the benefits you derive from them will be greatly enhanced if you eat them raw, lightly steamed (steaming cooks without leaching out nutrients) or lightly stir-fried. If you eat less than half of your vegetables raw or cooked in these ways, you are compromising the value of nutrients you're getting from them.

■ Do you store your oils in a cool, dark place?

Exposure to heat, sunlight and air causes the fats in oil to convert from less saturated, healthier forms, to more saturated, less healthy forms, and breaks down EFAs. If you answered no, you could be inadvertently lowering the quality of your fat intake. So don't keep your olive oil in a glass bottle next to your range cooker – find space in a cabinet some distance away. I buy mine in bulk, and pour it into a cool stone jar for everyday use.

■ What proportion of this week's food shopping was organic?

Modern methods of farming involve the heavy use of chemical fertilisers, highly toxic pesticides and herbicides, hormones, antibiotics and sometimes unnatural animal feeds in order to 'force' higher yields of crops and animals. The price we pay for this farming system is that our soils are increasingly depleted of minerals, and the food we eat often arrives in our homes depleted of much of its nutritional value, even before it is processed – as well as being contaminated with substances that may harm rather than feed us. For example, plants grown in selenium-deficient soil will be selenium-deficient, and so in turn will the population eating these plants. You should be aiming to buy as near to 100 per cent organic as possible.

ORGANIC VS NON-ORGANIC

With less than optimal levels of nutrients, and far too many contaminants, food produced by modern intensive farming methods may not be the best choice. But is organic better? Organic farmers follow practices that sustain soil health and fertility; use fewer, carefully chosen and only necessary medications in animal rearing, and follow high standards of animal welfare; and employ primarily natural methods of controlling pests, weeds and diseases. The result? Vegetables, fruit and meat that are low on contaminants, and relatively high in nutrients. And it is also often fresher, as much of it is grown in the country where it will be consumed. This is why naturopaths put so much emphasis on eating organic – you get organically grown food that usually comes from a local producer and goes through a minimum of processing and handling. Otherwise you may be buying food that is not only non-organic, but may have travelled halfway round the world, shedding nutrients as it went.

These days organic food is easy to find in most supermarkets, but it is generally more expensive than non-organic food – and this is where the sceptics come in. They claim there is no scientific evidence that organic food is better for you , so we are being duped into paying up to 40 per cent more for a gimmick. But science says otherwise. A 1999 inquiry by the British House of Lords found that organic produce had lower levels of undesirable nitrates and more vitamins, while a 2000 study by the UN agency, the Food and Agriculture Organization, concluded that it contained lower levels of pesticides and veterinary drugs. Other research quoted by the UK's Soil Association found that most organic produce contains significantly higher levels of vitamin C, iron, magnesium and phosphorus. That may not seem like much, but it may mean the difference between getting the recommended daily allowance – or failing to.

As a naturopath I also believe that pesticide contamination in non-organic food may possibly be linked to the huge increase in the allergies, degenerative diseases, and possibly cancers we are now seeing. I also suspect that in cases where it is not detected, the reason may lie with inadequate testing methods.

There are two more important considerations that the sceptics cannot dispute. First, when you pay extra for organic food, you are being a responsible consumer and using your money to encourage holistic farming methods that are better for the environment, as well as good animal husbandry. Secondly, organic food often tastes better – surely a prime reason to buy it. (See the Useful Addresses section at the back of the book for places you can go for more information on this important subject.)

Don't be discouraged, however, if you can't find organic foods in your area. The improvements in your overall diet that I've described are the most important change you can make for a healthy, enjoyable future.

■ How many meals (including breakfast) did you skip over the last week?

If you live in a city and have a demanding job, you'll already be pressured; add in a heavy social schedule and/or childcare, and you may find your eating habits deteriorating. You may even think that skipping meals is a useful way to diet. But missing out meals, particularly breakfast, is a terrible dietary habit. With no breakfast, your blood sugar levels fall dramatically – and come mid-morning you will find yourself craving sugary snacks. A lot of my women patients eat very little during the day, as they are fearful of gaining weight. But by mid-afternoon they find themselves overwhelmed by hunger, which they'll eat in the most instant form available – chocolate, biscuits and so on. And these calories will be converted directly to fat around the middle.

A study at the Harvard Medical School found that breakfast eaters have half the risk of developing obesity and insulin resistance (see box), major risk factor for diabetes and heart disease, compared to breakfast skippers. Breakfast seems to have a magical ability to help with calorie control throughout the day, not least because just digesting and absorbing food burns calories. But carb loading at night, say, by people who eat a big plate of pasta before going to bed, causes us to lay down fat. In studies, breakfast skippers who've been put on a breakfast eating plan have lost weight when they were previously unable to.

WHAT IS INSULIN RESISTANCE?

When someone eats too many refined carbohydrates (white bread, cakes, sugar and so on) or binges on them periodically, they subject their blood to sudden floods of glucose. This in turn upsets the balance of insulin (the hormone that carries glucose into muscle cells for use as energy) and may eventually trigger a resistance to its action. More glucose will remain in the blood, upping the risk for type 2 diabetes; and there will be more excess glucose to go into storage as fat.

One reason people miss breakfast is that they're simply not hungry enough when they wake up. If they ate very late the night before, they may still feel slightly full. I advise people to eat within an hour or so of getting up in the morning. If you're getting up too late to do this, take a healthy portable breakfast to work with you. Fresh fruit, yoghurt, homemade low-sugar granola, or maybe oatcakes are good choices to help you avoid the Danish pastries in the coffee bar. Limiting late-night suppers will also help you feel raring to go – and healthily hungry – in the mornings (see below for other reasons to go for an earlier evening meal).

A BETTER BREAKFAST

Beware of the hordes of breakfast snacks out there being marketed as portable and 'healthy'. They often contain huge amounts of sugar, and all that will do is give you a burst of energy, then a slump – and a craving for more of the stuff. Go for 'slow-burn' complex carbohydrates/low sugar snacks (oatcakes, or yogurt, fruit and a few oats and nuts are ideal).

If you skipped more than one meal in the last week, and especially if you make a regular habit of it, you could be causing yourself all sorts of dietary headaches.

How late do you eat dinner?

The timing of meals affects the way you metabolise your food – eat just before you go to bed, for instance, and more of the calories you've consumed are likely to be laid down as fat. If you ate not long before you went to bed several times during the week, it probably means you've got into a habit you need to get out of.

How many minutes did you take to eat your lunch?

In this busy world, even when we take the time to eat lunch, we may not take enough. Do you scoff your meals at your desk, trying to cause as little disruption to your work as possible? Do you hastily grab a sandwich and wolf it down so you can rush back to the office? Eating should be a leisurely process during which you have time to chew each mouthful and digest each meal. But more than that, mealtimes provide a vital moment of 'you-time' – a chance to change your surroundings, concentrate on something other than work and give your system a respite from stress. It is important to separate activities. Choose whether you are going to eat, work or watch TV; don't automatically snack when you sit down in front of the box, for example.

> **CHEW THIS OVER . . .**
>
> Think about whether you are really chewing your food properly. It has to be mixed well with saliva if you are to digest it fully. A sign of the times: a recent study found that the average McDonald's meal was consumed in less than 10 minutes in the US but over 20 minutes in France, where it seems ingrained to take time over any meal no matter what its content.

Could you have extra nutritional requirements?

In theory, anyone eating a balanced diet should be getting all the micronutrients they need, but in practice a surprising number of people may suffer from very slight but important deficiencies without realising it. One problem is that comparatively few people genuinely eat a balanced diet.

Another problem is the issue of food quality and modern farming methods, which we looked at earlier.

The deficiencies I'm talking about might not be recognised as such by a conventional doctor, because they fall short of the narrow clinical definition of the term. In the context of overall health, however, they can be significant, draining the resources you need to fight off infections or adding to the cumulative stress on your system. A slight change in diet leading to a very minor deficiency could prove the 'exciting cause' that triggers an illness.

WHY ARE YOU AVOIDING THAT?

Out of every 50 patients I see, 15 to 20 are avoiding certain foods, believing this will benefit them because of books or magazine articles they have read, rather than on any strict medical guidance. It's good to avoid fatty, sugary and salty processed foods. But there may be no good reason for you to avoid dairy foods or wheat products, and doing so may be to your detriment.

Groups who may be more at risk of micronutrient deficiency include children and the elderly; women who are pregnant, breastfeeding, taking the Pill or menstruating; or anyone who is drinking alcohol regularly and not eating well (very common), smoking, is a vegan or vegetarian, suffers from a malabsorption syndrome such as coeliac's disease, is on some form of (often self-imposed) exclusion diet, or is recovering from illness or injury. They may have a greater demand for certain micronutrients because of their condition, or because their diet is likely to be poor. People whose diet is lacking variety and/or quality are also at risk. If you are in any of these categories, you may want to think about taking appropriate supplements (see pages 60–1).

■ Do you suffer from any symptoms of micronutrient deficiency?

The following are all typical of the often non-specific health problems that micronutrient deficiency can cause.

- Symptom: recurrent mouth ulcers
Deficiency: iron, B vitamins, for example B12, folic acid

- Symptom: cracking at the corners of the mouth
Deficiency: iron, B vitamins, for example B12, folic acid

- Symptom: sore tongue
Deficiency: iron, B vitamins, for example B12, folic acid

- Symptom: red, greasy skin on your face (especially on the sides of your nose)
Deficiency: B vitamins, zinc or essential fatty acids (EFAs)

- Symptom: rough, sometimes red, pimply skin on your upper arms and thighs
Deficiency: vitamin A, carotenes, or EFAs

- Symptom: scrotal or vulval itching
Deficiency: zinc or EFAs (should also check for diabetes)

- Symptom: rough skin conditions such as eczema, dry, rough, cracked, peeling skin
Deficiency: zinc, EFAs

- Symptom: poor hair growth
Deficiency: iron or zinc, EFAs, B vitamins

- Symptom: bloodshot, gritty, sensitive eyes
Deficiency: carotenes, vitamins A, EFAs

- Symptom: night blindness
Deficiency: vitamin A

- Symptom: brittle or split nails
Deficiency: iron, zinc or EFAs

- Symptom: white spots on your nails

Deficiency: zinc (though they can also be caused by trauma to the nails, for example while typing)

- Symptom: pale complexion

Deficiency: iron, vitamin B12, folic acid

If you suffer from symptoms like this, or a combination of them, and your GP's investigations can find no clear cause, deficiencies may be a likely culprit.

All about micronutrients

Minerals and vitamins

Sub-clinical micronutrient deficiencies – ones that a doctor might not recognise but that can still cause health problems – are surprisingly common. One way to tackle deficiencies is through supplements, and we'll discuss these. Ideally, however, your diet should meet all your micronutrient needs, and following some simple rules can help to ensure that it does.

- Eating a diet rich in vegetables, especially leafy green vegetables like spinach and kale, dark-green cruciferous vegetables like broccoli and cabbage and dark red berries and tomatoes, will provide lots of beta-carotene (which your body converts into vitamin A) and vitamin C.

- The most common deficiencies are of iron and zinc. Iron-rich foods include meat, eggs, beans, shellfish, parsley, nuts, green vegetables and wholemeal bread. Combine them with vitamin C-rich foods – vitamin C helps to increase iron absorption in the gut. Don't overboil your vegetables as this decreases their nutrient content radically. Some foods decrease iron absorption, such as tea, coffee, bran and unleavened bread (such as chappatis), which are rich in phytates – part of the fibre content of wheat that is broken down in the process of leavening bread, but remains in unleavened bread (and is known to inhibit calcium, iron, zinc and probably magnesium absorption). People who eat phytate-rich foods every day are at risk of iron-deficiency anaemia, and should take precautions. Rich sources of zinc include fish, shellfish, eggs, ginger, most types of nuts, peas, garlic, carrots, turnips, beans and corn. Zinc absorption can be impeded by soya-based foods, alcohol, laxatives, tea and coffee and many types of medicinal and recreational drugs.

- Eat nuts and seeds. They are rich sources of practically all the micronutrients (seeds are especially good for essential fatty acids or EFAs) but all too rarely feature in the average diet. To make delicious snacks, mix several types together. Ones I particularly recommend include pumpkin, sunflower and sesame seeds, and pine and pistachio nuts, and I always have a bowl of these on the side in my kitchen for the family to dip into. Some people find seeds hard on their teeth. Try soaking them in yoghurt, water or juice to soften them up, or grind them in a coffee grinder and add them to cereal or salads. Seeds that are not properly chewed or ground up will not release their oils, so the nutritional value is not obtained (they were, after all, designed in the food chain to go 'in one end and out the other', as animals ate the seeds and then in due course distributed them by excreting them!). A lot of patients proudly tell me they regularly eat linseeds or sesame seed snaps. These are a valuable fibre and bulking agent, and can have a laxative effect because they lubricate the digestive tract, but it's the oil you need for nutritional benefit. Small seeds such as sesame and linseed are hard to chew effectively and so their oils are not readily released, so grind them wherever possible.

- Red meat is a rich source of many micronutrients, so if you're not eating it you need to make sure that you compensate for its absence. Of course this particularly applies to vegetarians and vegans, who are at high risk of some mineral deficiencies such as iron. Variety is the best way to compensate for the reduced meat consumption – eat as wide a selection of seeds, nuts, eggs, pulses, grains, fruits and vegetables as possible.

- Calcium is essential for strong bones and particularly important for postmenopausal women, growing children and teenagers, pregnant and breast-feeding women, the elderly, vegetarians and those on exclusion diets (see Chapter 6). Dairy produce is one of the richest sources of calcium, but people who want to reduce the amount of fat in their diet needn't despair: skimmed milk and low fat dairy products have very little fat content but plenty of calcium. One pint of semi-skimmed milk provides 690mg of calcium (compared with 660 in full fat milk), roughly half an average adult's daily requirement. Ensure good calcium absorption by increasing the amount of vitamin D in your diet – good sources are oily fish (such as sardines – a good source of both calcium and vitamin D) and cod liver oil. If you get enough calcium throughout your life, you'll help keep your bones strong and protect against osteoporosis in later life. Osteoporosis is a particular risk for people who follow or have followed fad diets or who are chronically underweight – and for teenagers who may tend to eat particularly erratically and drink a lot of fizzy drinks (which contain phosphates, which increase the excretion of calcium via the kidneys and cause a net calcium loss). We reach our peak bone mass around the age of 25, so building strong bones in childhood and young adult life is vital for the future.

Antioxidants

Vitamins and minerals play a number of roles in your metabolism; one of the most important is as antioxidants. Antioxidants are 'housekeeping' molecules that mop up damaging free radicals – highly reactive toxic agents produced both by normal metabolic processes and as a result of pollution, exposure to UV light, smoking and so on. Free radicals are believed to play a part in ageing, cancer, arthritis, coronary heart disease and other degenerative diseases, so antioxidants are vital for health. Vitamins A, C, E and beta-carotene and the minerals selenium and zinc are powerful antioxidant micronutrients supplied by your diet, and, once again, fruits, vegetables, nuts and seeds are the richest sources. A good dietary tip for cutting down your intake of free radicals is to avoid barbecued, charred, reheated, bruised, burnt food or smoked foods, and preservatives and additives – basically anything that is not completely fresh or is past its sell-by date.

Do you need supplements?

If you ask your GP whether you need supplements, you will probably be told that unless you are a special case (for example, iron deficient) all your nutritional requirements should be met by 'a balanced diet'. The trouble is that, as I have explained so far, most people do not have a sufficiently varied and high-quality diet. Added to that, they are unlikely to get all the necessary advice about this from their time-starved GP.

So should you go for supplements? There are a number of pros and cons. First, it should be said that the supplements industry is worth billions, and that plain ignorance about nutrition and fear of ill health leads many to waste an awful lot of money on capsules, pills and potions they simply do not need. Some of my patients arrive in my clinic with A4 sheets listing all the supplements they are buying after consulting one therapist or another (who will no doubt be making a neat profit from the purchases).

Secondly, there is also a lot of debate about the issue of how well micronutrients are absorbed and utilised by the body when taken in supplement form. Some opponents of supplements go so far as to claim that they are largely useless, and that your body is unable to access all but a tiny percentage of nutrients taken in this form. This is almost certainly an exaggeration, but it is definitely true that you are better off getting your nutrients from whole foods where possible.

And if you are following the kind of diet I am advocating, and are in generally good health, you will almost certainly be getting enough micronutrients. Although research on the relative efficacy of supplements and whole foods in delivering nutrients is ongoing, whole foods are still better for a number of reasons.

- Whole foods typically supply a wide range of nutrients at once.

- Micronutrients in whole foods arrive in your digestive system in forms different from the ones you get in supplements. They may be easier to absorb and utilise in these forms, although this is not certain.

- Micronutrients in whole foods come in combination with each other, and also with a range of other substances, many of which have not been studied, and whose function so far remains mysterious. There is, however, evidence that this combination helps to increase the absorption and utilisation of the nutrients in your digestive system.

- Whole foods are generally much cheaper than supplements.

Deficiencies   So far, so good – as far as whole foods go. The question is, do they go far enough in every case? National nutritional surveys show (and the personal experiences of many naturopaths and nutritionally trained doctors back this up) that surprising numbers of men and women show deficiencies in zinc, magnesium, iron, calcium, folic acid, some B vitamins and EFAs. Conventional medicine often misses these deficiencies because they occur at a sub-clinical level – that is, they don't produce the clear-cut signs of deficiency described in the textbooks, such as scurvy or beri-beri – but a range of micronutrients might be involved. And today's deficiencies are more likely to contribute to chronic illnesses, fatigue, mental health problems and depressed immune systems than scurvy.

Doctors are also often misled by the notion of recommended daily allowances, or RDAs. Many RDAs have been set at fairly arbitrary levels, and probably fail to match the needs of many people. For example, the UK's RDA for vitamin B6 was set following a study on dogs, not humans, and the results took into account the 'uncertainty factor' – that dogs of all shapes and sizes may be taking the vitamin – so the average was set to cover every permutation. If we were to assess people for micronutrient deficiencies with blood tests we would find widespread sub-clinical deficiencies.

And for some people, deficiencies are serious enough for them to need a considerable boost in micronutrients. This may be indicated if either their intake is very low for some reason, or their requirements have gone up for some reason. You should consider taking supplements, or at least talking to your healthcare adviser about it, if you fall into one of the following groups.

- Children and young adolescents experiencing growth spurts, and the elderly; women who are menstruating heavily, on the Pill or just coming off it, planning a pregnancy, breastfeeding, or undergoing the menopause; and alcoholics, smokers and drug users. All these groups have increased micronutrient requirements – either because of natural processes such as ageing or growth, or self-imposed physical stress such as smoking – and a normal diet simply may not meet all their needs.

- Vegetarians, especially vegans, and people on restricted or exclusion diets, because their diets are more likely to be deficient in micronutrients. Vegans are particularly at risk of vitamin B12 deficiency.

- People who live alone (often, again, including the elderly), the bereaved or depressed are more likely to be on a poor, monotonous diet deficient in micronutrients.

- People who are ill or recovering from illness that has put extra demands on their system. Also, if you suffer from chronic or recurring low-level illness, including depression, skin problems or fatigue, nutrient deficiencies can either be contributing to them or make them harder to shake off.

- People taking medication.

Unless your deficiency is serious and obvious, or your healthcare adviser says otherwise, you should always try using food sources to boost your micronutrient intake for one month or so before you start taking supplements. Not only will you be more likely to get the most out of your extra micronutrients, you'll also improve your diet, probably boost your fibre and antioxidant intake and save money. And if you find you do need to take supplements, bear these considerations in mind:

- If taking medication, check with your doctor first. Some drugs and supplements can interact with each other. For example, you should not take essential fatty acid or vitamin E supplements if you are also using blood thinning drugs, as they have a similar effect.

- For some supplements, caution is advised for pregnant women or those planning to get pregnant – particularly with vitamin A, which has been linked to birth defects.

- Check your supplements, especially ones bought from chemists or supermarkets, for tartrazine and other additives that can aggravate allergies, and also for substances such as sugar, yeast, wheat, gluten, milk/lactose, corn, soya, artificial additives or sweeteners like aspartame which may affect some people adversely. The best supplements are additive-free, except for the gel capsule or a binding agent or two.

Deciding what to take   Diagnosing specific micronutrient deficiencies can be hard and may require expert consultation and blood testing. I find, however, that the supplements I most commonly prescribe are for the minerals zinc, magnesium, iron, calcium and selenium.

- **Zinc** is one of the supplements I prescribe most often. It's only needed by the body in minute quantities, but is important for immune function, healthy bones and skin, for healing, for the nervous system, and for sexual function. Do not take zinc long-term without nutritional advice, though, as it can interfere with the absorption of other minerals.

- **Magnesium** is another. You need magnesium for muscle and nerve function and particularly for a healthy metabolism. The risk of deficiency is high because processed foods – such as white bread, junk food and alcoholic beverages – are particularly poor in magnesium.

- **Iron** is needed to maintain healthy blood and to carry oxygen around the body and to our muscles and brain. It's also important for nervous system function and hair and nail health. Again, deficiency may be more widespread then is commonly recognised, particularly among women of childbearing age, and especially those with heavy and prolonged periods. Other groups at risk include pregnant women, growing children, people recovering from surgery and those eating a limited diet, such as the elderly or depressed. Look for a supplement that provides 8.7 to 14.8mg. Don't take iron supplements with tea, coffee or foods containing bran – take them with fruit juices or other vitamin C sources. It's vital not to over-supplement with iron; see the box below.

AVOID IRON OVERLOAD

It is important to stress that it is possible to oversupplement with iron, which can lead to 'iron overload' – the deposition of iron in the liver and soft tissues. Men and postmenopausal women (who aren't losing blood through menstruation) are particularly vulnerable. In my practice I see probably two cases of iron overload each year that are caused by supplementation. In extreme cases this can require venesection – taking off a unit of blood each month until the iron overload is resolved.

- **Calcium** is vital. For people who have trouble meeting their calcium needs through dietary intake, such as vegans, those who are intolerant of the milk sugar lactose, and those avoiding dairy products for health reasons, supplements may be necessary. The average daily requirement is about 1000mg, but this increases to 1500mg for women over 45. When buying a calcium supplement, check the level of available calcium it provides, rather than the total amount of calcium salt. For instance, 1000mg of calcium carbonate contains only 400 mg of available calcium – the rest is carbonate salt. Don't take more than 1000mg per day.

- **Selenium** is often overlooked. You only need 60 to 75 micrograms (mcg) of it daily, but this mineral is important as an antioxidant and for your hormonal and reproductive systems. Research suggests that selenium levels in the soil are dropping, increasing the general risk of deficiency. Look for a daily supplement that provides about 50 micrograms. Again there are risks of selenium toxicity, so do not double up, for example by taking one multivitamin and mineral supplement and another for antioxidants that both contain selenium.

MINERAL-RICH FOODS

You can take supplements for all the minerals I've mentioned. But it's just as easy getting them from some very tasty foods . . .

- Half a dozen oysters will provide 30mg zinc; muesli and sardines are less concentrated sources.

- 2oz (60g) of almonds, brazil and cashew nuts or a bowlful (5.2oz or 150g) of muesli will provide nearly 150mg magnesium.

- 3.5oz (100g) dried apricots provides 5mg iron, and the same amount of liver provides 9mg iron.

- 4oz (120g) whitebait or one and a half pints of milk will provide 1000mg calcium.

- Five freshly shelled Brazil nuts will provide 100mcg selenium.

If you do need a supplement you will maximise its absorption and minimise your risk of side effects if you follow these simple rules:

- Take supplements after a meal, unless otherwise directed.

- Wash them down with water or fruit juice. Taking an iron supplement with vitamin C-rich fruit juice enhances its absorption.

- Avoid taking them with tea or coffee, especially iron, zinc or magnesium supplements.

- If you have trouble swallowing a supplement, look for special, coated easy-to-swallow types or chewable ones. Dissolvable calcium supplements are also available, which is useful as calcium tablets are usually large. Your doctor or pharmacist can advise about this.

- Take supplements separately from medication.

- If taking a general or multivitamin supplement, get one that is not time-released. In the UK, follow Food Standards Agency directives unless there is a specific need for higher levels of supplementation for a defined period.

- If taking various supplements, spread them out during the day.

Side effects and adverse reactions are possible, especially with high doses. Common examples of side effects are:

- Taking large amounts of vitamin C will cause stomach irritation or loose bowels.

- Taking large amounts of magnesium can cause diarrhoea. This is understandable, as the well-known laxative, Epsom salts, is in fact magnesium sulphate.

- Zinc can cause stomach irritation and nausea.

If side effects do occur, stop taking the supplements and check with your doctor. Reintroduce them one by one, in smaller doses. If they were causing digestive problems take them with meals. Note that B vitamins can cause your urine to go bright yellow, but that this is quite harmless.

HEALTHY EATING PLUS

- Variety is the key to a healthy diet

- Poor quality food cannot deliver the full range of nutrients we require

- Many minor but common health complaints may be caused by micronutrient deficiencies

- Appropriate supplements are worth considering as an adjunct to your diet if you're vulnerable to deficiencies for reasons such as age, physical conditions such as pregnancy, illness or depression

CHAPTER 6

Allergies and intolerances

About four out of 10 of my patients are afflicted with minor but persist ent problems such as digestive upsets, headaches, joint pain and bad skin. Such symptoms come and go, niggling at the edges of their health and happiness. And for many of them, allergies, intolerances and sensitivities are contributing factors.

These conditions are being reported in the media a lot these days, and it's sometimes hard to make sense of it all. One of the biggest problems is that there's a lot of disagreement about what is and isn't an allergy.

An allergy is a condition in which inhaling, eating or sometimes even simply touching a trigger substance produces an allergic reaction. Antibodies in the sufferer's system recognise part of the trigger and set off an allergic response that may manifest as swelling, difficulty breathing, rashes and/or itching. A typical example of a serious allergy is peanut allergy, which is a well-known cause of potentially fatal anaphylactic shock. The mechanisms of this type of reaction are well understood and generally easy to recognise, and you will certainly know if you or someone in your family has this kind of allergy.

Intolerances (or sensitivities) to certain substances are much more contentious. Sufferers may be sensitive to more than one food, for instance, or to an ingredient common in many foods. Any one trigger – say, wheat – may produce different symptoms in different individuals. In one person it may trigger migraine, in another abdominal symptoms, and in another, nasal congestion. Intolerance can also manifest as chronic fatigue, gut disorders or eczema. The range of symptoms is huge. Moreover, the mechanisms that underlie some allergies are poorly understood, and it is often hard to distinguish them from non-allergic reactions or unrelated illnesses.

INTOLERANCE AND SENSITIVITY

Intolerance and sensitivity are widely used terms, but are generally poorly defined or understood. Strictly speaking, an intolerance is where your body (usually your digestive system) lacks the necessary tools to deal with a substance (usually a component of food), which does not get properly broken down/digested and thus causes problems. A classic example is lactose intolerance. The digestive system of people with this condition lacks the enzyme lactase, which is needed to break down lactose, a sugar found in milk and dairy products. Lactose then arrives undigested in the lower intestines, resulting in bloating and disturbed bowel function.

'Sensitivity' is a term used to describe a reaction to a substance where the mechanism/cause isn't fully understood. A relatively common example is chemical sensitivity, where simply smelling a trigger chemical causes symptoms such as migraine or nausea.

Do you suffer from chronic symptoms but can't find out what's causing them? How can you work out whether an allergy is to blame? Allergic symptoms may not appear to be linked to any particular trigger substance, but even intolerances follow some general rules.

■ Signs and symptoms of allergies and intolerances

- Do you have four or more of the following symptoms? Fatigue or low energy levels; poor concentration; dry skin/eczema; painful joints; susceptibility to thrush infection; excessive wind; bloating; feeling tired after meals; anal itchiness.

- Do you suffer from any chronic symptoms of varying severity that your doctor has had little success in diagnosing/treating despite medical investigations and/or referral to a specialist?

- Do you suffer from a combination of symptoms? For example, more than one of the following: eczema, migraine, IBS, asthma or hay fever.

- Is there a pattern to your symptoms? For example, do they worsen after meals or after certain types of food; do they worsen at certain times of the month or year; are they linked to a particular area or part of your house/workplace? Is there something that relieves them (such as visiting the sea or mountains)?

- Have you ever been advised to exclude foods such as chocolate and cheese (tyramine-rich foods) for migraine? Or to try a hypoallergenic diet such as the Stone Age Diet? If so, what were the results?

- Have you ever kept an allergy diary, noting what you have eaten and when, along with symptoms such as rhinitis or tickly nose, and other possible triggers (dust, for example)?

■ Are you suffering from four or more unexplained symptoms?

If you find yourself suffering from fatigue or low energy levels, poor concentration, dry skin/eczema, painful joints, susceptibility to thrush infection, excessive wind, bloating, feeling tired after meals or anal itchiness, you may have an allergy or intolerance. But these symptoms can also be a sign, when accompanied by abdominal symptoms, of a condition known as fungal type gut dysbiosis. This is discussed fully in Chapter 11.

■ Do you suffer from chronic symptoms of varying severity that your doctor has had little success in diagnosing/treating?

Symptoms caused by intolerances tend to be chronic and persistent, but may vary in severity over time. Because the link between trigger and symptom is hidden and the symptoms themselves tend to be hard to pin down, doctors find it hard to correctly diagnose causes and often can do little more than treat symptoms.

■ Do you suffer from a combination of symptoms, such as eczema and irritable bowel syndrome, poor concentration and migraine?

Multiple, apparently unrelated symptoms can be a classic marker of intolerances, even if a conventional diagnosis/treatment has been given for each one individually. Eczema coupled with irritable bowel syndrome (IBS), or fatigue coupled with migraine, are good examples.

One poor man who came to see me was literally the colour of a boiled lobster. His face couldn't have been a brighter red and he was hugely embarrassed by it. He had seborrhoeic eczema with a flaky scalp and flaking skin around his hairline and across his face. He also had the symptoms of IBS, and these flared up when he ate piping hot or sugary foods, and wheat. The link between this type of eczema (which tends to be greasy, yellow and scaly) and IBS is well recognised by naturopaths, and a change of diet to ease his extremely uncomfortable gut problems and improve his general wellbeing happily also solved the embarrassing problem that had eroded his confidence at board meetings and in social situations. He was hugely thankful, and I was very pleased. As an added bonus, he no longer required the steroid creams that would have slowly aged and damaged his skin.

■ Do your symptoms follow a pattern?

By comparing the pattern of your symptoms with an overall picture of your diet, habits and environment, you might be able to pick up clues about allergic causes or triggers. The obvious example is seasonal rhinitis (hay fever), where the worst symptoms will tend to coincide with pollen release from certain species of plant. Perennial rhinitis (which affects sufferers all year round) is often linked to dust mites – if symptoms are worse in the mornings on waking up, it is a sign that dust mites in your bedding and pillows may be to blame.

Geographical variation in symptoms may also be a clue. I once had a patient who realised that her illness (a mixture of chronic fatigue and irritability) came on most strongly when she walked through the perfume and cosmetics area of a department store or was exposed to cleaning products, suggesting that she was chemically sensitive. If symptoms improve during a trip to the sea or mountains, this might suggest that the causes lie at home – perhaps the trigger is something to do with your house or office (a sign of the so-called sick building syndrome), or the pollution levels of your town or city. A lot of patients tell me they feel worse at work. For more about sick building syndrome, see page 174.

Finally, allergic symptoms are often made worse by stress, or become more severe at certain times in the menstrual cycle.

■ Have you tried a hypoallergenic diet?

Hypoallergenic diets such as the 'Stone Age' diet are specifically designed to eliminate some or all of the foods that most often trigger food intolerance reactions (see Chapter 7 for more information). Lots of people have tried a diet like this as part of a detox programme, or maybe while attending a health spa. If you've ever followed one for more than four days, your reaction could provide a valuable clue to the origin of any unexplained symptoms you suffer.

If your symptoms improved as a result of following a diet like this it strongly suggests that a food allergy or intolerance is to blame. Bear in mind that it can take up to two weeks for symptoms to improve, so a negative result right at the start doesn't rule out an allergy or intolerance.

Believe it or not, feeling worse while on such a diet also shows that you might have been on the right track. Withdrawal symptoms are a common feature of hidden allergies. Successfully cutting a trigger food out of your diet can cause tiredness, muscle aches, headaches, nausea and weight loss, typically lasting for three to five days. Most people I treat have had some experience of this – if only the classic 'weekend headache' caused by withdrawal from the usual high volumes of coffee and other caffeinated drinks they consume while at work.

■ Have you ever kept an allergy diary?

An allergy diary is an extended version of the food diary you've been working on. It provides one of the best ways to find out, for yourself, whether you are suffering from an allergy; but it does require patience and attention to detail.

On each day for at least two weeks you have to record everything you eat and drink, including all the ingredients of processed foods. Some food additives, like gluten or powdered egg, can be common hidden food allergy triggers. At the same time you must record all symptoms, together with their severity and the time of day they are better or worse. You also need to record information about your weight (sudden weight gain due to water retention can be a symptom of hidden food allergy), bowel habits (when you open them and the nature of your stool – see page 131 for guidance) and any medications you are taking.

If you have kept an allergy diary, bear in mind that it can take an expert eye to discern patterns in the diary, particularly if your symptoms are caused by intolerance to more than one foodstuff. Ask your GP for a referral to a hospital allergy clinic, or find a registered naturopath (see 'Resources' at the end of this book). In the UK they must have the letters ND MRN after their name.

There's a growing concern among doctors and environmentalists about how chemical residues and additives in foods may themselves react with each other and influence our own biochemistry and health. As humans, we are all biochemically similar, but not identical, so we may react individually to chemicals in our food or indeed to the 'chemical soup' that surrounds us, possibly developing a range of symptoms individual to ourselves. The action of some chemical additives mimics that of hormones, which may also affect us. Some people with severe chemical sensitivity can develop a wide range of debilitating symptoms such as rhinitis, headaches and fatigue. They may undergo a number of medical tests to discover the root of their problems, but many will emerge from these with no known cause and the same old symptoms – often feeling, sadly, that their doctors believe them to be malingerers.

It's not unusual for such sufferers to be referred for counselling or to a psychiatrist. This is no criticism of conventional GPs – but we do need to broaden our knowledge in this area. The symptoms themselves can be a significant cause of low mood. But in some cases depression and mood swings can be triggered by the intolerance. This is not yet generally accepted by the medical profession but I am certain research into nutritional psychiatry will in time reveal some underlying mechanisms.

ARE YOU REALLY INTOLERANT?

Some people are genuinely intolerant of some foodstuffs or food groups, and may benefit from medically supervised exclusion diets. Too many people, however, are excluding certain foods from their diets when they're not actually intolerant of them – wheat and dairy products being the most common examples. If you suspect that you suffer from a food intolerance, follow these simple rules:

- Don't totally exclude foods without a clear reason for doing so – that is, after a proper nutritional/medical evaluation indicates that this may be a valuable management plan.

- Consider the deficiencies that may result from your exclusion, and make sure you eat alternative sources of the missing nutrients. An example is dairy exclusion – you'll need to top up your calcium requirements from other foods.

- Don't ever apply an exclusion diet to your children without medical advice.

Pinning down an intolerance

If you suspect you have a food intolerance and want to pin it down, what's the best exclusion diet? In my opinion, it's the Addenbrookes Diet, which we'll look at now.

Named after the Cambridge hospital where Professor John Hunter and his colleagues devised this regime, the Addenbrookes Diet is a tried and tested version of an exclusion diet for avoiding the majority of foods to which a person may be intolerant. As a rule, exclusion diets are extremely tricky but the

Addenbrookes is one of the best and easiest, making it the most popular. In my opinion people following this diet should do so under medical supervision (that is, they should have guidance from an appropriately experienced doctor before, during and after the diet and food reintroduction phases). Any risk of serious reaction to a food must be evaluated and advice given.

The Addenbrookes Diet

- Hunter advises keeping a food and symptom diary for three days before starting the diet, so your progress can be judged.

- Once you've begun, stick to the diet strictly for two weeks.

- Your doctor needs to monitor withdrawal symptoms over the two weeks. The most common include headaches, nausea and abdominal discomfort.

- In addition to the listed foods, avoid any that you already suspect of being triggers.

- Foods should be eaten fresh or frozen, and organic wherever possible.

- Avoid all tinned, packet or convenience foods.

- Some symptoms may worsen before they improve, but stick to the diet regardless. After two weeks, consult your doctor if there's no improvement – perhaps food allergy or intolerance isn't the problem! If not, then you can reasonably exclude them, and explore other possibilities.

Addenbrookes Diet dos and don'ts

Food	OK	Don't eat
Meat	All fresh meat	Preserved meats, bacon, sausages
Fish	White fish, oily fish	Smoked fish, shellfish
Vegetables	Green vegetables, salad, tomatoes, pulses, beans, peas, lentils	Potatoes, onions, sweetcorn

Food	OK	Don't eat
Fruit	Apples, pears, bananas and non-citrus fruits	Citrus fruit
Cereals	Rice, ground rice, rice flour crisped rice, rice cakes tapioca, sago, millet buckwheat	Wheat (including bread, cakes, biscuits, pasta, noodles), rye (crispbreads), oats, barley, corn (including cornflour, corn on the cob, gravy mix, custard powder), breakfast cereals (except crisped rice)
Cooking oils	Sunflower, safflower, soya and olive oil	Corn or 'vegetable' oil
Dairy produce	Soya milk, goat's or sheep's milk, yoghurt or cheese	Cow's milk (including dried milk, whey, casein, lactose), cream, butter, yoghurt or cheese
Beverages	Pure water, apple, pineapple and tomato juices (fresh), alcohol, herbal teas	Tea, coffee, fruit squashes, citrus fruit juices
Other	Sea salt, herbs, spices in moderation, sugar, honey	Chocolate, nuts, vinegar, yeast and yeast extracts (Vegemite, Marmite) preservatives

Sample menus

- Breakfast: Buckwheat porridge with dried fruit or crisped rice and soya milk, apple juice, rice cakes

- Lunch: Meat/fish, rice, vegetables/salad, fruit or soya milk pudding

- Dinner: Meat/fish, vegetables/salad, fruit or goat's milk yoghurt.

Reintroducing food This is the phase when food reactions may occur, and reintroducing foods *should not be attempted without medical supervision.* Most reactions reproduce a person's original symptoms, such as migraine or abdominal problems, but severe reactions are also possible.

Here's what you do. When your symptoms have cleared, reintroduce the banned foods one by one in the order listed below. Keep a food and symptom diary. Try each food for two days, and if symptoms do not return, move on to the next. If symptoms do return, discontinue that food and wait for at least two to three days before testing any new food, as your symptoms may linger.

Foods should be reintroduced in the following order, in a very strict regime. You don't want to undo all the work you've already put in. After two days without reaction, you can include that food in any of your meals:

1. Tap water

2. Potatoes

3. Cow's milk

4. Yeast (take three brewer's yeast tablets or 2 teaspoons of baker's yeast in water)

5. Tea

6. Rye – if yeast test was negative (rye crispbread or rye bread, checking that there is no added wheat)

7. Butter

8. Onions

9. Eggs

10. Oats

11. Coffee

12. Chocolate (plain)

13. Barley (add some pearl barley to a soup or stew)

14. Citrus fruits

15. Corn (cornflour or corn on the cob)

16. Cow's cheese

17. White wine

18. Shellfish

19. Cow's milk yoghurt (natural, not flavoured)

20. Vinegar

21. Wheat (shredded wheat first or try wheat flakes)

22. Nuts

23. Preservatives (such as those found in fruit squashes, tinned food, sausages, smoked fish and so on) – even though I generally advocate a fresh food diet, it may be useful to know by dint of this reintroduction process whether these preservatives are affecting you in any way. MSG and saccharine should be last of all, although I urge you not to bother reintroducing them!

ALLERGIES AND INTOLERANCES

- *Seek professional help if you suspect an allergy or food intolerance. Do not embark on self-diagnosis and treatment*

- Most people know if they are genuinely allergic to something. An intolerance is harder to define and diagnose

- A huge number of symptoms can be linked to intolerance

- Keeping a symptom diary will help you identify problems and their triggers

---

CHAPTER 7

The McManners Method Diet

B y now you may have guessed that I do not believe in faddy diets and am not going to boss you into adopting one. Instead, I encourage variety and quality in what my patients eat, and I believe there is no 'one size fits all' diet for health. So, you may be asking yourself, how can I now advocate a McManners Method Diet? Am I not about to lead you into just the kind of regime you've seen a hundred times before? Hopefully not. What I want to give you are the means to make your own optimum diet.

To explain how I have arrived at my dietary advice, here's a brief lesson on the history of nutrition.

Many people believe that the dietary transition we've undergone in the last 200 years is to blame for modern Western health problems. The theory is that modern methods of farming and food production have reduced the fibre in most of our diets while introducing more protein, refined sugar, salt, fat and artificial additives and contaminants than would ever have been available to our ancestors in pre-Industrial times.

Other experts go further back, blaming changes that took place 10,000 years ago, in Neolithic times, when hunter-gatherer communities were beginning to settle and develop methods of farming. According to this theory, to which I also subscribe, the human digestive system evolved over millions of years to cope with a hunter-gatherer diet that changed very slowly over time. But since the Neolithic era, the rapid pace of change within agriculture, food processing and technology has altered our diet too quickly for the process of evolution to keep pace – so now we are eating a diet we're not really designed to digest and use with ease.

Both these theories imply that at one time mankind lived in a sort of nutritional Golden Age, eating an ideal diet that ensured optimum health, and that modern humans have fallen from grace, at least in the kitchen. The truth, of course, is far more complex. Overall, we're far more healthy and live for longer now than our pre-Industrial or Stone Age ancestors, and in many ways the average present-day diet may be far superior to theirs. But there is also much we can learn from the way our ancestors ate when we are trying to determine a good model for a healthy diet, because at their best they shared a number of important characteristics:

- **Less meat**: opinions differ on the prevalence of meat in the Stone Age diet, but it seems likely that for much of the time meat was scarce. Crucially, when people ate it, it was wild food – game, which is generally considered to be better for our health.

- **More fish and seafood**: as people tended to settle near water, fish and shellfish were more common protein sources.

- **Unprocessed food**: the absence of modern processing and manufacturing meant that there was much more fibre in the diet, whole foods were more prevalent and sugar and salt were very rare indeed. Before the introduction of sugar refined from sugar cane, for instance, the only sweetener available to Europeans was honey, and this was a rare luxury.

- **Uncontaminated food**: all ancient farming methods were what we would call organic, as artificial fertilisers and pesticides hadn't been invented.

- **Fresh food**: the absence of refrigeration or preservation methods meant that a lot more of the diet had to be composed of seasonal fresh food, although this also meant that fresh foods were scarce at some times of year.

- **Combination with lifestyle factors**: people were generally more physically active, and were not exposed to modern toxic pollution.

FASTING FOR HEALTH

Our ancestors probably did not eat plentifully every day and were the healthier for it. Some days, when they had killed a deer or large animal, they ate a lot of meat over a two-day period (before the carcass went off). Other days, particularly when out hunting, they expended vast amounts of energy without obtaining any food. Human physiology evolved to cope with – and thrive on – this pattern of food consumption, but today we eat more than enough food at practically every meal.

While I generally advocate eating regularly and not skipping meals, I am also aware that fasting or semi-fasting can be energising and may help the body to ward off illness. I tend to recommend a semi-fast – for example, a day of fruit in the morning, fruit or vegetables at lunch and vegetables in the evening, with plenty of water or diluted juice to drink throughout the day. I sometimes also encourage a weekend semi-fast of two to three days, during which you drink only fruit and vegetable juices (but plenty of them, and always diluted 1:1 with water) on the first day, adding steamed vegetables on the second, and seeds and grains on day three.

To avoid a detox headache, build up to a semi-fast by eating light, healthy foods for a couple of days beforehand and avoiding coffee, cigarettes and other stimulants. Don't eat a heavy 'last meal'. (I remember being at a naturopathic clinic and spotting a woman eating a huge 'family size' pack of chocolates before she drove through the gates. Not the best way to start!) During your semi-fast, try to avoid eating dinner out at a restaurant or at friends' houses, as fasting just isn't compatible with people enjoying gourmet feasts. If you have a partner, try to fast together. Despite being a very natural activity, any degree of fasting should be treated with care. You have to take it easy as you will have much less energy during it than usual. Keep warm, exercise gently such as taking walks outdoors and take relaxing baths. And drink lots of water – at least 2 litres a day.

Best of both worlds: pesco-vegetarianism

My favoured model for a healthy everyday diet is one that takes into account the general rules outlined above. Technically, it might be called a pesco-vegetarian or pescatarian diet – a mainly vegetarian diet but with fish and other seafood included as sources of protein and other important nutrients (especially zinc and EFAs, in which many people are deficient). Most of the fish should be of the oily, EFA-rich variety, especially trout, herrings, sardines and wild or organic salmon.

The main bulk of a pesco-vegetarian diet is made up of basic complex carbohydrate sources: lentils, beans, couscous, wild rice, millet, quinoa, wholemeal pasta and wholemeal bread, together with lots of fresh fruit and vegetables, and a good variety of nuts and seeds. The majority of meals should be essentially vegetarian, though not slavishly so – unless you're a vegetarian for ethical reasons, of course. Remember that the guiding principle should be variety.

Fish might figure several times a week – perhaps some mackerel in a salad at lunchtime, or some fish in a stir-fry at dinner – but again, it's the overall spirit of the diet that's important, not the details. Flexibility is key, and you should feel free to pig out occasionally. Eat ice cream or order a pizza every now and then; eat whatever your friends are serving at their dinner party; enjoy the occasional barbecue. As long as your overall diet is a healthy pesco-vegetarian one, you'll be building nutritional and vital reserves aplenty, and your system won't be troubled by the occasional less healthy meal (so you'll avoid irritating friends by making things difficult for them).

The main benefit of a pesco-vegetarian diet is that it's tasty, enjoyable and easy – and, of course, incredibly healthy without an ounce of 'worthiness' in sight. Such a diet provides a good balance of food groups, which matches up well with official food pyramid guidelines. It is low in saturated fat, sugar and salt, high in fibre, rich in all the vitamins, minerals, antioxidants and EFAs, and provides all the essential amino acids. It is quite likely that humanity's historical diet would have been mainly pesco-vegetarian, both in pre-Industrial and Stone Age times.

> **CHILDREN AND VEGETARIANISM**
>
> Giving children a vegetarian or mainly vegetarian diet requires special care. Either get professional advice from your doctor or dietician, or get in touch with a group like the Vegetarian Society (see Resources), who can offer sound advice on the subject.

Getting used to a new dietary style takes time. You should ease into it gently. Begin by eating one pesco-vegetarian meal a day. Take the time to experiment with new ingredients and new recipes, and don't get too bogged down with the rules. As Socrates said, 'Everything in moderation. Nothing to excess.' In other words, avoid lifestyle extremes.

> **KITCHEN ESSENTIALS**
>
> The healthy kitchen doesn't require a lot of expensive gadgets. The three key pieces of equipment in my kitchen are:
>
> - A large steamer for fish, vegetables and couscous
>
> - A large sauté pan – essentially a large stainless steel frying pan with a lid; ideal for preparing ratatouille and dishes like dahl, and stews of pulses and beans
>
> - A terracotta baking brick for fish, meat and game
>
> I would also advise investing in porcelain or stainless steel cookware, to rule out the risk of introducing aluminium, a toxic heavy metal, into your food.

Good digestive habits

As I've said before, it's not only what you eat that's important, but how you eat it. The pioneering naturopaths of nineteenth and early twentieth century Europe placed a great deal of emphasis on good eating, and the need to reform their patient's habits. Sometimes this was taken to comical lengths – Dr Franz Mayr, who devised the so-called Mayr Cure in Austria, advocated chewing as the route to internal happiness, insisting that 'only things that taste better after being chewed 50 times are good for you'. As exaggerated as this seems, there was also a lot of truth in their advice. Let's take a look at some of the principles of healthy eating.

- **Eat regularly.** Regularity is vital for healthy physiological function, which can affect everything from your mood to your intelligence. Children who eat breakfast, for instance, perform better at school than those who don't. Never skip meals (except when you're undergoing a fast, as outlined on page 81).

- **Breakfast like a king, lunch like a prince and dine like a pauper.** This is one of my favourite dietary maxims. It reminds us that most people have their meals the wrong way round (in terms of size). The start of the day is when you need a good launching pad of energy and nutrients, with a secondary boost at lunchtime. Yet most people eat the biggest meal of the day in the evening, shortly before sitting around relaxing and then going to bed. As someone once observed, 'The engineer does not stoke his engine before putting it in the shed for the night.' The end of the day is when your metabolism is winding down. Your digestion is less efficient and excess calories are more likely to be laid down as fat, while the lack of physical activity means your intestines will have less help in pushing food through your digestive tract. Big meals just before bedtime can also disrupt your sleeping patterns.

- **Eat more frequently.** If tailoring your meals so breakfast is bigger than dinner is problematic, try breaking up your food intake into smaller but more frequent meals – every three hours or so.

- **Eat more slowly.** Eating on the run or under stress does your digestive system no favours. Mealtimes should be calm. You'll enjoy your food more too. Take positive steps to relax, even if you don't have a great deal of time. Sit down to eat, and try to leave the office for a change of scene.

- **Chew your food.** Dr Mayr may have been slightly over the top on mastication, but it *is* a vital part of the digestive process. Without the mechanical break-up of food, especially the more fibrous plant foods that compose the bulk of a healthy diet, the rest of your digestion is labouring at a disadvantage. Chewing also helps to mix your food with lots of saliva, which contains the digestive enzyme amylase that kick-starts carbohydrate digestion in the mouth. So don't wolf down your food in great chunks (which also tends to make you swallow air, as well as preventing full digestion).

- **Stop when full.** According to Austrian naturopath Erich Rauch, an ancient Egyptian physician observed, 'Most people eat too much. They thrive on a quarter of what they eat and the physicians thrive from the other three-quarters.' Today many people still eat more than they need, ignoring the simplest, most basic signal that tells them when to stop – when they feel full. Make this a cardinal rule of your eating – stop when you feel full. Avoid making more food than you're going to need, and don't finish a dish for the sake of it.

- **Improve your bowel function.** Eating more fibre is the best way to do this, but you should also drink lots of water (see below), try to visit the toilet at a regular time each day and never ignore a signal to go to the loo. Straining is bad – it probably means that you need to eat more roughage and drink more water. Chewing and eating more slowly are also helpful.

- **Water, water, water.** Water is essential to life, health, good digestion, clear skin and a generally healthy appearance. You should aim to drink 2 litres or so a day (more in a hot climate or when you're exercising hard). You may find it hard to boost your fluid intake at first, but make the effort. Your urine should be clear and odourless – if it's not, you're not drinking enough.

STICKING TO YOUR NEW REGIME

- Always have breakfast. Missing it may cause you to eat more later.

- Plan your meals ahead, so that you've got recipe/menu ideas for a week in advance. This will help you to do the shopping for your new diet, and lessen the chances of your slipping back into old habits for the sake of convenience.

- Make sure you have the right foods in the house, or you are more likely to end up eating the wrong ones. If you don't buy biscuits, ice cream and so on, you won't be tempted to snack on them.

- If you are hungry between meals, have a snack, but make it a nutritious one, such as low-fat yoghurt, fruit, seeds or cereal.

- Never go food shopping when you're hungry.

- Make a shopping list and stick to it.

- If you eat out, explore different culinary styles, and use your meals as research for inspiration you can take back to your kitchen.

- Think about why you are changing your eating style. A healthy diet will increase your chances of good health now and in the future, and improve your energy levels and appearance.

- Remember: 'all things in moderation'. In other words, eat chocolate and drink beer sometimes if you want to – just don't overdo it. And don't eat lima beans if you don't like them – there are plenty of other healthy foods that you will like.

- Be adventurous. Explore new cooking traditions. I've already suggested Mediterranean and Middle Eastern cooking, which are both delicious and healthy. Japanese cuisine also has a lot of low-fat, tasty fish and vegetable meals (sushi, for example); and South American cookery features unusual grains like millet and quinoa. Cookbooks covering every cuisine under the sun stuff bookstore shelves, so have a go, and use the recipes as an inspiration for your own variations and inventions.

- Get into the healthy eating habit. Many healthy eating techniques seem difficult at first, but only because we've learned unhealthy habits. In practice, couscous and a bean, fish or game stew are as easy to make as a cream-laden curry; steaming veg is as easy as deep-frying them; and you quickly get used to having less salt with your food.

> • Be creative when you're shopping and cooking. Always be thinking about how you can add variety to your diet and replace less healthy foods with equally tasty and convenient healthy ones, instead of feeling deprived of foods that you're not 'allowed' to have.

Making it work

Most people find it helpful to stick to some kind of a routine. Especially while you are getting accustomed to your new style of eating, it may be useful to refer to a list of healthy main meals you can rotate every 10 days or so. Try the following or come up with your own menus.

1. **Ratatouille:** chop Mediterranean vegetables – peppers, aubergines, tomatoes, onions, garlic and courgettes – and sauté slowly in a dash of olive oil, serving with cracked wheat.

2. **Paella:** sauté small quantities of organic chicken with fish, shellfish and vegetables (onions, peppers and peas), then add brown or wild rice seasoned with garlic, saffron and chilli and chicken or vegetable stock, and cook without stirring till rice is tender.

3. **Salmon:** grill simply and serve on a bed of Puy lentils tossed with wilted fresh spinach, seasoned with lemon juice.

4. **Fish with chickpeas:** grill or steam white fish and serve with chickpeas cooked in a spicy tomato sauce (cook the chickpeas, or use a drained tin of them, and add to homemade tomato sauce seasoned to your liking with herbs or spices such as cumin and ginger).

5. **Wild meat:** roast venison, partridge, pheasant or wild boar and serve with dahl – a thick 'porridge' of orange lentils with onions and spices.

6. **Vegetable stir-fry:** stir-fry a multicoloured medley of vegetables (try carrots, bok choy, green onions, fresh ginger, French beans and red peppers and finish off with a big handful of spinach leaves, just allowing them to wilt), and serve with rice.

7. **Sardines (fresh grilled, or tinned):** serve with couscous or tabbouleh (couscous mixed with chopped peppers, onions, nuts, dates and herbs and served cold) and salad.

8. **Cauliflower cheese:** serve with flaked white fish and baked potatoes.

9. **Slow-cooked vegetables and pulses:** choose root vegetables and cook slowly in a casserole with tomatoes, spices and a handful of cooked chickpeas and haricot beans, served with wholemeal bread, brown rice or wholemeal pasta.

10. **Mackerel:** grill and serve with rice and vegetables or salad.

Working lunches often present a problem. But you don't have to rely on the nearest sandwich bar! I work in London twice a week, and take my own lunch with me – usually fruit that I buy at the railway station, seeds, oatcakes, yogurts, and maybe even a cold baked potato with a filling or a slab of cold fish and a sliced avocado with lemon juice in a Tupperware box. Cold falafel patties with salad leaves and ripe tomatoes, or a wholewheat pasta salad with olive oil dressing, a hard-boiled egg and plenty of chopped raw vegetables, are easily packable and nutritious, too. And if you're pressed for time or forgot to bring anything, some lunch outlets have now got the message and are offering excellent salads, a choice of rye or other low-wheat breads and healthful toppings for the ubiquitous baked spud.

This might be enough of a guide for you, but some people find it helpful to get specific instructions for new diets. I usually provide patients who ask for them a sheet outlining menu ideas and allowed foods. Below you'll find detailed advice on everything you need to know to formulate a basic healthy eating/weight loss diet.

The healthy eating/weight loss diet

This pesco-vegetarian diet aims to reduce your calorie intake, boost your micronutrient intake and avoid unhealthy foods.

Breakfast options

- A glass of vegetable juice, a piece of fruit and two oatcakes.

- Yoghurt and millet flakes, with a piece of fruit.

- Wholemeal toast topped with a grilled tomato and olive oil, baked beans, one boiled or scrambled egg, or 2oz (about 60g) sautéed mushrooms.

- My real favourite is porridge – half to one cup of organic oats soaked overnight in soya or semi-skimmed milk and then heated. You can add fruit or seeds – whatever you fancy. This really fills you up and hunger pangs shouldn't strike until lunchtime.

Lunch options

- A large baked potato topped with a low-fat cheese, sweetcorn or tuna mixed with onion, peppers or olives, with lightly stir-fried vegetables or a salad.

- A large salad, either green or with cold rice, with 3oz (85g) trout, mackerel or other oily fish. Use a dressing made with about a tablespoonful of cold-pressed olive oil, and a big pinch of fresh or dried herbs.

- A large bowl of vegetable soup, ideally homemade, with a chunk of wholemeal bread (try breads made from different grains – oat and rye are good).

- A sandwich with egg, cheese, fish or avocado and lots of salad – try various combinations of tomato, lettuce, julienne carrots, beansprouts and cucumber – and pine nuts.

- Thick wholemeal toast drizzled with olive oil and topped with olives and sundried tomatoes.

- A quick ratatouille (see page 87).

Dinner options

- Fillet of fish, such as salmon or a whole trout or sole, with plenty of green vegetables or salad and, optionally, 4–6oz (110–170g), cooked weight, of wholewheat pasta, brown or wild rice, millet or quinoa.

- Vegetable stir-fry or casserole with a small amount of oil, on a bed of brown rice, couscous or cracked wheat.

- Spiced tofu (or a fillet of oily or deep-sea fish, as above) served with curried lentils.

Snacks
- Oatcakes, olives, nuts and seeds, crudités, yogurt, half an avocado, hummus.

Food allowances and cooking instructions

- **Fish:** cook by grilling, baking or steaming. I sit mine in a little water in a stainless steel pan in the oven so they don't stick.

- **Fried foods:** ideally none, or stir-fry with a minimum of oil.

- **Oils and fats:** use small amounts of pure vegetable oils, preferably cold-pressed.

- **Bread:** stick to wholemeal – try all varieties of grains.

- **Pasta and rice:** try to use wholewheat pasta or newer types made with rice, corn or other grains, and brown or wild rice.

- **Fruit:** eat at least three pieces a day, preferably fresh. If tinned, go for varieties packed in unsweetened fruit juice; and limit the amounts of dried fruit you eat.

- **Vegetables:** use fresh vegetables, cooked in a minimum of water or steamed. Don't add salt – old habits die hard, but you need to wean yourself off it. Doing without salt will re-educate your palate and then you'll notice the subtle flavours of the food.

- **Eggs** (a great source of protein, lecithin – a vital brain food – and minerals, as well as omega-3 fats in varieties from specially fed chickens): boiled, poached or scrambled. Omelettes are also excellent, and quick.

- **Milk, cheese and yoghurt:** use lower fat varieties (such as skimmed milk and Gouda cheese). Go for live bio yoghurts made with acidophilus cultures to ensure healthy gut flora.

THE MCMANNERS METHOD DIET

- Go for pesco-vegetarian menus

- Be adventurous in your cooking

- Enjoy your food

- Don't skip meals, but consider the occasional semi-fast – juices and a light vegetable diet for a day or two

- Pay attention to how you eat

- Make healthy eating a creative challenge

CHAPTER 8

Healthy living

June, one of my regular patients, came to see me after a gap of some months. She had been well, more or less – there was nothing obviously wrong with her. But she did feel tired, lethargic, with vague headaches that seemed to come on more at home, and also since the change to autumnal weather. Quite a few of my patients come in with a wide variety of undefined symptoms. In fact, hospital consultants seem to make a point of referring such patients to me for an in-depth assessment of all the factors that may be influencing what's actually going on.

Many of these people have already undergone extensive investigations to exclude important underlying disease. The results might all have been negative, but the patients still feel ill. But discovering what's really going on doesn't involve magic. It involves looking at the bigger picture: the environment that person lives and works in.

I begin by taking a detailed history of the person's contact with their environment, and the kind of things they may be exposed to, such as dust and chemicals. We look at factors such as:

- Their job

- Where they work

- Whether they live on a busy road

- Whether they live in a basement flat

- The pattern of their symptoms, and whether there is any relation to possible toxic load or chemical exposure.

I examined June, and carried out some investigations, but these failed to reveal any clues. We talked at length about the environmental aspects of her workplace and home. In the end I asked her to have the gas appliances checked and serviced – which should be done in every home at least once a year.

She came back to tell me that the engineer had found her gas central heating boiler to be leaking carbon monoxide. The boiler was repaired and her symptoms resolved. She thanked me and I was very pleased the problem had been identified. Carbon monoxide is a hidden problem in many homes, and can be lethal. There has been some publicity about it, but nowhere near enough to heighten public awareness of this dangerous hazard in the home.

So, alongside your own health checks, give your house a health check to make sure it's a healthy environment for you and your family. In practice, a healthy home works together with healthy eating – as they are, after all, the two elements of biochemical health.

Lucy came to see me on account of abdominal pain, bloating and fatigue after meals – all signs of IBS. She said that she actually felt better if she did not eat. Lucy lived an incredibly busy life as a DJ, wife and mother, and had already made changes to her incredibly demanding schedule so she could keep relatively regular hours; but her abdominal problems persisted. To compound the issue she also suffered rhinitis – a constantly running nose, like all-year-round hay fever – and her sleep (not to mention her husband's!) was disturbed by her snoring.

I asked her to follow a naturopathic dietary regime and to make changes in line with my guidelines for a healthy house. This involves house dust mite avoidance and eliminating chemical cleaning agents, sprays, chlorine compounds and so on, from the home. The effect was hugely beneficial. First, her energy levels improved: renewed vitality is always very welcome and a good sign that things are improving generally. Better still, her IBS settled completely and so did her rhinitis. She felt so well, in fact, with her renewed energy that she's having another baby!

Lucy's story underlines the fact that it's vital to pay full attention to your internal environment, especially diet; and to your external environment; in this case exposure to allergens and chemicals in the home.

If you think you have a few areas of concern in your own home environment, don't despair. There is nearly always something you can do to improve matters, though the changes you may have to make could range from the simple to the drastic. At one end of the scale are things like leaving the lids on pans of boiling water to limit condensation and the growth of moulds. At the other end are wholesale life changes like moving house (and even neighbourhood) or finding a new job. How far you need to go depends, of course, on how badly your health is affected.

■ Looking at where you live and work

- Do you live on a busy road? Describe the levels of traffic fumes in your local area:

    Heavy   Moderate   Light

- Are any of these present in your local area? Power station, incinerator, factory/plant, landfill, train/ship handling facilities, fields, crop-spraying, woodland, damp or marshy areas (bottoms, dells, valleys and so on).

- Which of these are present in your home/work environment? Double-glazing, central heating, wall-to-wall carpets, deep-pile carpets, metal window frames, unventilated shower, washing machine/tumble dryer not vented to outside, or MDF fittings and furnishings.

- What pets live with you (cats, dogs, rodents or birds)? Do they come indoors or live outdoors only? Are they allowed in the bedroom?

- Is your house damp, and if so, how do you deal with it?

- In your house, how often do you vacuum, and what type of vacuum cleaner do you use? (Does it have a HEPA filter, recommended for allergy sufferers?) How often do you wash bedding and soft furnishings, and at what temperature? Do you regularly scrub mould and deposits from bathroom, shower, fridge, windows and so on?

- Do you have a gas cooker or other gas appliances?

- Do you use air fresheners, fabric/carpet fresheners, deodorants, perfumes, polishes, bleaches, cleaning products, photocopiers or printers? Are any of the following present in your home/ work environment: new synthetic building materials, freshly painted/treated surfaces/walls, cavity wall insulation, ceiling tiles?

- Is there any smoking in your house?

- Is there a switching station, electricity pylon, high-voltage power line, mobile telephone mast within a quarter of a mile of your home? Do you use a mobile phone? Have you ever checked out the websites for different phones to find out which gives the lowest level of emissions?

Sensitivity to environmental factors such as these can vary hugely. I've dealt with cases of such extreme chemical sensitivity that the sufferers found it difficult to hold down a job, and cases of perennial rhinitis so bad that the sufferer could hardly get a decent night's sleep. People in the throes of this kind of health problem are often desperate to get back to some sort of normal level of health and are ready to take drastic steps. But in quite a few people, the harmful effects of pollution and allergens may not show up as a specific condition. Their impact on your health is more to do with their effects on your overall toxic and allergic load, and the cumulative effect of individual environmental influences.

In this chapter, I'll show you how to lighten this load and relieve some of the pressure on your system. Radical life changes may not be practical, but small changes can have a positive cumulative effect. By helping your immune system you'll lessen the drain on your reserves and can start building them up instead, to counteract the forces that are throwing your health triangle out of kilter.

■ How bad is the traffic where you live?

Obviously, traffic fumes and smog are generally worse in urban areas than rural ones, and in some cities compared to others. Diesel fumes are probably the most dangerous type of traffic pollution, as they contain diesel particulates – toxic particles that can burrow deep into your lungs. But petrol fumes and emissions from cars add to outdoor pollution levels, which have been linked to rising rates of asthma. Move to a back bedroom if possible, or use an air purifier.

■ Are there other sources of pollution in your neighbourhood?

Power stations, landfill sites or incinerators generate air pollution (such as sulphur dioxide emissions and sooty particles), which can be particularly bad in areas with poor air circulation, such as low-lying land, narrow valleys or places encircled by hills. They can also affect the water supply. A recent report revealed significant chemical load in fish near the Queen's Balmoral estate. Other potential pollution hotspots may be less obvious – if you live near a port, for instance, you could be at risk of exposure to high levels of diesel emissions from ships.

People in rural areas are not always better off in terms of this kind of pollution. Extensive use of chemical sprays in agriculture has been linked to many health problems, while contamination of food and groundwater by fertilisers and pesticides is a hazard that affects all of us. Is there much spraying in your area? You can check the health of your water supply by getting in touch with the local water company who should be able to tell you, month to month, whether the water in your area is within EC and British guidelines for allowed limits of chemical compounds.

Allergens can come from natural sources as well as artificial ones. Seasonal rhinitis – also known as hay fever – is often linked to the pollen of a particular plant. Allergists can use 'pollen calendars' to work out which one is likely to be triggering hay fever in a sufferer. In the UK grass pollens, which come into season in May, June and July, are the most common hay fever allergens. In the US it's ragweed pollen, which is in season in late summer. Tree pollens typically cause problems in February or March.

Mould spores are much less well known as allergens, but may be present in higher levels than pollen. Even at the height of the grass pollen season there are around 50 times more mould spores in the air than pollens, adding greatly to the allergenic load on your immune system. Warmth and humidity accelerate mould growth, and spores are most prevalent in late summer and autumn, and in wooded and/or damp, sheltered areas, cellars and basements (see below). The spores can cause the same sort of health problems triggered by pollen.

■ Is your house an indoor pollution trap?

Asthma and other respiratory problems are getting more and more common, but it's not only outdoor pollution that's to blame. Asthma rates can be higher in rural areas than urban ones, while hay fever is a worsening problem in urban areas despite overall falls in the levels of airborne pollen in cities – evidence of the problem of indoor pollution and of the interactions between chemicals and allergens.

Indoor pollution is made up of two main categories: natural sources such as house dust mite droppings and moulds, which can be extremely allergenic, and chemical pollution, which can be toxic (see page 108). Your home may have features which could be increasing your exposure to both of these.

Saving on energy, losing on health

During the fuel crisis of the 1970s, many homes introduced energy-saving measures to cut their fuel bills: double-glazing, draughtproofing and insulation. Many of these features are now standard in most new houses as part of the move towards energy efficiency. But are smaller fuel bills a good enough reason to foster conditions that may be a real risk for our health?

Sealing up our houses in this way makes them warmer, less well ventilated and more humid – all conditions that favour the growth of house dust mites and moulds, two of the biggest contributors to allergy. One only has to see the condensation from our breath on sealed windows early in the morning to understand how it increases humidity. High levels of house dust in the home have been linked to respiratory illnesses and certainly increase the allergenic and toxic load on the people living there.

House dust mites are tiny lice-like insects that feed on discarded flakes of human skin. They thrive in moist, warm conditions and particularly in the deep pile carpets and soft furnishings and beddings that so many of us now prefer. Dust mite droppings, together with parts of dead insects, are extremely allergenic.

The same conditions that favour dust mites also encourage the growth of moulds, especially in poorly ventilated households where people take lots of showers, cook with open pans, have metal window frames that encourage condensation or use air conditioners, washing machines and tumble dryers without proper outlets. The common black aspergilla moulds that grow in bathrooms and on the seals of refrigerators produce spores that are toxic, allergenic and carcinogenic. Indeed, a frightening array of pathogenic organisms will grow on the average shower curtain, so ideally these should be put through a weekly hot wash.

Basements, generally being damper than the rest of the house, are also breeding grounds for moulds. Don't have your bedroom in the basement if you can help it, and think seriously about where your children are sleeping in the house too. One of my patients developed chronic rhinitis after moving to a beautiful 'luxury' conversion flat bought for her by her parents, advertised as being on the 'lower ground floor'. This was just estate-agent speak for 'basement flat' and, despite its lovely appearance, whenever she returned from a weekend away she was aware it smelt rather damp and musty. Her symptoms resolved when she moved. If she had been unable to move, installing a dehumidifier – which takes out water from the air, so discouraging mould growth – would have helped. (See page 101 for information on dealing with dust, dust mites and mould.)

▪ Do you have pets – and do they live indoors with you?

Many animals – including cats, dogs, hamsters, gerbils, horses, rats and mice – can trigger or exacerbate allergies. The triggers can include urine, dander (hair and skin flakes) or particles of cat saliva (cats clean themselves with their tongues – the saliva dries and flakes off, producing one of the most pervasive and persistent household allergens). For some people, just entering a room where a cat has been sleeping can trigger sneezing, itchy eyes or asthma. I recently saw a woman who developed an itchy rash on her neck and forearms after cleaning a carpet in her newly rented flat. The key was its history. The previous tenant used to allow a cat into the flat, and even though this was months before, she was still very badly affected.

Pets produce allergen 'hotspots' in parts of the house where they live or play. If you allow pets into your bedroom and other living areas, you are significantly increasing your allergenic load. Pets do us a lot of good, and can be wonderful companions, especially for isolated or elderly people, but allowing a dog or cat the free run of the house isn't the best option for some susceptible people.

■ How damp is your house, and how are you dealing with it?

We've seen how damp and poor ventilation can allow dust mites and mould to proliferate. Now let's look at how you can combat the demon damp in your home – as well as the nasties that breed with its help.

Dampness is the scourge of the allergic, and the enemy of all those who want to make their homes as healthy as possible. As we've seen, house dust mites and moulds depend on moisture for growth and reproduction, while low humidity levels slow down the growth of mould and stop house dust mites from breeding.

None of us can escape dampness. Remember, we're made up largely of water, so it's inevitable that our dwellings will feel the effects. Each of us gives off around 2 pints (over a litre) of water every day at least, including about a pint a night in the bedroom – much of it into your pillow and mattress, where dust mites love to congregate. More moisture comes from cooking and washing (especially showers). Then there's all the water trying to get in from the outside, through our floors, walls and roofs, via precipitation and atmospheric moisture, as well as damp from the ground.

There are four major strategies for reducing moisture levels in your home:

1. preventing its initial appearance

2. helping it to get out once it's got in

3. cutting down on condensation

4. removing moisture from the atmosphere artificially.

Down with damp

1. **Prevention** Probably the best way of avoiding moisture is prevention, rather than cure.

    - If you're moving house, choose a dry site. Avoid houses sited *very* close to water, in deep hollows or other sheltered areas or closely surrounded by trees. Check with local authorities to see whether flooding has been a problem in the area.

    - Tackle structural problems. Leaky pipes, rising damp due to faulty damp courses, leaky roofs and the like can let water into your house from outside. Correct structural defects and invest in a good damp course, but try to avoid ones based on potentially irritating chemicals. Alternatives include electro-osmotic damp-proofing or hollow clay tubes. Also be careful how you treat rising damp or dry rot – synthetic pesticides may cause more problems than they solve, and emissions from them may seep into the air for years. Use treatments based on water-soluble borates.

    - Cut down on day-to-day sources of humidity. Think about domestic activities that cause humidity. Put lids on pots and pans of boiling water; consider taking baths instead of showers; keep the door of the bathroom/kitchen shut while washing/cooking and ensure you have adequate ventilation (I always open the window slightly); dry your washing outside or use a tumble dryer vented to the outside. Remember that gas heaters create moisture.

2. **Improve ventilation** Ventilation is another vital issue. A poorly ventilated home with double-glazing, draughtproofing and all the features of the modern home is, as we've seen, a moisture trap. And poor ventilation doesn't just exacerbate dampness; it also prevents the escape of chemical fumes and vapours so that they are more likely to build up. Here's how you can let in some fresh air to dispel the damp.

    - Leave windows open or ajar where possible, especially in your bedroom at night and in the bathroom or kitchen while showering/cooking. Obviously this rule doesn't apply if the air outside is going to cause worse problems than the air inside – say, during summer for hay fever sufferers, or if you live on a busy road.

- Make sure that the bathroom and kitchen are fitted with extractor fans, but remember that they need an air inlet somewhere else such as an open window, or they won't work.

- Install trickle vents around windows so that moist air is constantly escaping.

3. **Cut down on condensation** Condensation is a huge problem in some homes. Here's how to deal with it.

- Wherever moist air meets a cold surface the moisture will condense to give the sort of conditions that moulds love. Identify the damp spots in your home and keep those areas as warm and dry as possible.

- Mop up condensation on windows or wall tiles with a cloth, and then dry it outside.

- Don't use mattresses with plastic covers. Moisture will condense on the inside of the cover.

4. **Dehumidify if you need to** Sometimes rooms such as basements demand extra help if they're not to feel like a temperate rainforest. Dehumidifiers can do the trick.

- Keep the atmosphere in damp rooms warm and ensure the ventilation is as effective as possible.

- Use a dehumidifier – extra-powerful ones are available for damp-sensitive people, who may develop rhinitis or headaches in places like basements.

■ Is your cleaning regime effective against dust mites and mould?

You don't have to remodel your house or do away with all your carpets and double-glazing to deal with house dust and dust mites. Fortunately, there are other ways you can tackle the problem directly and lighten your allergenic/toxic load. You'll need to vacuum regularly and with the right equipment – ideally, a vacuum with a HEPA filter that will reliably remove fine particles. And you will have to complement your cleaning with tougher steps such as washing your bedding in hot water, and scrubbing mould hotspots like shower and bathroom tiles.

As a general rule, the dustier your house, the more dust mites you are likely to have. Dust mites, as we've seen, eat flakes of cast-off skin (one of the major components of house dust) from humans or animals, so anywhere or anything that has a lot of contact with people or pets is likely to be a dust mite hotspot. Below, you'll learn how to vanquish them.

Defeating dust mites

You can tackle dust mites in three ways:

1. preventing them from multiplying in the first place

2. attacking them directly

3. removing them and their allergenic debris.

1. **Prevention** Prevention, as always, is better than cure. Here's how to head the mites off at the pass.

   - Reduce moisture levels in the home as described above, including ensuring good ventilation, especially in the bedroom.

   - Keep dust mites out of your bedding. Fit your duvets and pillows with anti-mite covers – these have very tiny holes that let moisture out but prevent mites or their droppings from getting in or out. Duvets and pillows filled with hypoallergenic material are a good investment. Air your bedding every day to keep it dry, and do so in bright sunlight when possible. If you've had the same bedding or mattress for years, think about getting a new one.

   - Upholstered divan beds make good homes for mites. You'll be better off with a ventilated wood or metal spring bed.

- Mites love carpets – the thicker the pile, the better. Think about replacing carpets with wooden, cork or tile flooring, but be careful about treated or synthetic materials that may emit noxious fumes. Use washable cotton rugs with ventilated underlays to soften the floor.

- The more cluttered your home, the harder it will be to clean and the more dust will build up. In particular, avoid clutter in your bedroom or children's bedrooms – for instance, don't use underbed drawers, and don't store books and shelves of soft toys in the bedroom. Use washable curtains instead of Venetian blinds.

- Keep pets out of bedrooms and as much of the rest of the house as possible.

2. **Attack** If the mites have spread in your house and you're feeling the effects, you'll need to attack them directly. The creatures are sturdy and notoriously hard to kill (which is why prevention is so important), but there are a few things you can try.

- High temperatures (over 66°C) can kill dust mites. Wash bedding, pillows, rugs, curtains and especially pet bedding and children's soft toys regularly at high temperatures.

- Mites don't like low temperatures either – a good trick is to freeze things like pillows and soft toys (pop them into a plastic bag first) before washing them.

- There are several anti-mite pesticide treatments on the market, but tests show that they don't work very well, while the toxic chemicals involved can cause problems for sensitive people.

- Tannic acid treatment can make dust mite droppings less irritating (by 'denaturing' them), and can be applied to carpets and upholstery. It needs to be repeated every three months. The tannic acid dries to a fine powder which is then vacuumed away.

- To treat carpets and upholstery, you can buy or hire steam cleaners or get a professional in for liquid nitrogen treatment, which freezes mites to death but doesn't harm the furniture. Follow treatments with heavy vacuuming.

3. **Removal** Manual removal of the mites and their droppings really helps. Here's how.

- Dust with a damp cloth – feather dusters simply put dust in the air, worsening allergic symptoms.

- Vacuum regularly – several times a week – but don't use an ordinary vacuum cleaner because their filters tend to let mite droppings out and recirculate them into the air. You need to use a hypoallergenic vacuum cleaner with high-grade bags and special HEPA filters.

- Groom pets regularly to cut down on the amount of hair or dander they shed, but do it outside. Try using a vacuum cleaner attachment that sucks up the debris as you groom.

- Air filters can remove allergens circulating in the air, but again you need to make sure you've got a high-grade filter or it won't catch the real culprits. Look for HEPA (High Efficiency Particle Air) filters, which use minute glass fibres less than a thousandth of a millimetre thick to trap even the tiniest motes of dust. Alternative types of filter, like ionisers or electrostatic air filters, don't help much with allergenic particles.

Mastering mould

As you'll have gathered, the best way to discourage mould from growing in the first place is to reduce humidity levels in the home and avoid condensation. Try these methods for reducing mould, too:

- Don't allow food to become mouldy – keep a close eye on fruit in particular. If I notice any signs of mould I put it straight on the compost heap!

- Moulds love the damp soil of a pot plant. Either avoid indoor plants altogether, or cover the soil with a layer of pebbles or sand and water only from the bottom.

- Keep a close eye on mould hotspots like rubber seals around the fridge and the shower curtain and grouting. The black discoloration on these areas is mould. Clean them regularly, but use simple treatments that won't provoke chemical sensitivities – sodium bicarbonate and borax are two options. Borax also makes a good mould-retardant spray on problem areas. Hot wash and air your shower curtains regularly so they dry out between showers. The bottoms of the curtains are particularly prone to mould.

- Follow the same precautions as you would for tackling dust mites – use high-quality vacuum cleaners and air filters.

- Dust and damp aside, the other big source of indoor pollution is toxic chemicals. I discuss the different types below – and unfortunately, there are quite a few – before detailing how you can work towards a relatively chemical-free environment at home and at work, starting on page 108.

Are you exposed to toxic gases?

Some toxic chemicals emanate from cookers, boilers and ordinary household materials. Gas cookers, for instance, produce high levels of nitrogen dioxide – according to some studies, higher than those found in the worst traffic pollution blackspots – which is believed to play a role in sensitising people to other airborne pollutants. Other gas appliances, such as old gas boilers, can leak high levels of toxic carbon monoxide, as we've seen.

Cavity insulation, carpets, paints, furnishings and ceiling tiles give off chemical fumes in a phenomenon known as outgassing. This is where chemical molecules escape into the atmosphere as gas. Although the quantities that outgas are tiny cocktails of trace gases, they can produce serious health risks when acting together. In fact, a gas cooker alone can release as much nitrous dioxide as you'd get if you stood in the middle of a dual carriageway. Some people are sensitive to this, others are less so. Personally, I feel sick and develop a headache near gas.

■ Are you exposed to volatile organic chemicals?

The other major type of chemical pollution your house is likely to harbour are the volatile organic chemicals (VOCs) that are found in all sorts of ordinary household subtances – cleaning agents, polishes, deodorants, antiperspirants, air fresheners, perfumes, detergents, waterproofing treatments, toner and photocopier/printer inks, decorating materials and some processed woods, fibreboards and glues.

Even trace amounts of VOCs can trigger symptoms in sensitive people. Their effects on the rest of us are not properly understood, but they almost certainly increase toxic load. And over the last 50 years there's been a huge increase in the chemicals to which we are exposed. Levels of VOCs may be 15 times higher in houses less than three years old compared with houses three to 18 years old; and more than 800 volatile organic chemicals were detected when studying the air quality within four US buildings in one study (see the box for an extreme example of this problem, and what one man had to do to overcome it). Many of these are xenobiotics – completely synthetic compounds that do not occur naturally and certainly are not naturally found in us – and they need clearing from our bodies. This process depletes crucial enzymes, and you need to redress the balance in your body by ensuring that you're eating a high level of micronutrients in your diet.

'MY NEW APARTMENT'S GIVING ME A HEADACHE!'

Nick was a young investment banker – a direct, no-nonsense chap, the sort who normally hasn't got the time for minor illnesses and believes that people suffering from fatigue need to 'pull their socks up'. Despite this, he was plagued by exactly the sort of symptoms he was would normally dismiss out of hand – vague headaches, lack of concentration, 'brain fog', a stuffy nose, wheezing and lethargy. He felt especially terrible in the mornings, and was worried about his work performance, as his concentration seemed to be impaired.

Investigations, blood tests, and a chest X-ray all failed to show any problems, so after taking a full history and talking about his diet and general lifestyle, Nick and I discussed the environment in which he lived

---

and worked. He'd recently moved into a brand-new flat in a completely renovated building in central London, dropping him slap-bang into a domestic environment rich in insulation products, fibreboard, solvent glues, paint and new carpets – all sources of volatile chemicals.

Worse still, tardy builders had delayed Nick's moving in. After several months of lodging with friends, he had been desperate to get into his own flat and had moved in as soon as he possibly could – only to hit the peak outgassing period for all those new materials, when they were giving off the most chemicals. This is a common problem for people who move in hot on the heels of builders and decorators.

With the problem diagnosed, and given the state of Nick's health, his only solution was to move out. Luckily, serendipity intervened and he was able to leave for a six-month posting overseas. His symptoms resolved while he was away, and in his absence, the flat vented itself of most of the allergenic chemicals. It was fortunate that Nick had been able to take this drastic course of action, because in cases like these there is a risk of developing sensitivity, where even very low levels of the chemicals involved can trigger symptoms.

■ Is there any smoking in your house?

Pretty much everyone knows about the health risks of smoking, passive and direct. What's less well known is that cigarette smoke lingers in fabrics and furnishings around the house and office, and the 4000 chemicals it contains re-emerge over time to add a nasty cocktail of toxic gases and cancer-causing particles to indoor pollution.

■ Are you exposed to electromagnetic pollution?

Electromagnetic (EM) pollution is a controversial issue, but I have dealt with many patients who appear to be sensitive to EM fields; and I have had personal experience of the problem in a house where I used to live. When we moved in, everyone noticed that one room in the house, nicknamed the 'slow room', seemed to have a peculiar atmosphere that made one feel dopey or groggy. It later turned out that the major power line ran into the house just outside the room. So living or working in the vicinity of a phone mast, power lines or other major source of EM fields might well add to the burden on your system.

What you can do about toxic chemicals at home and at work

There is a lot you can do to combat chemical pollution at home and in your workplace, and in this section I give you a range of tips on how to cut out sources of chemicals and chemical vapours. These are environments you have some say over. But in many cases, there's not much that you as an individual can do directly to reduce some of the more obvious forms of pollution. With problems like traffic fumes, agrochemical spraying and waste incinerator or power station fumes, the best thing you can do is to avoid them. This might mean changing your route to work, keeping your windows shut, altering your daily routine to avoid peak emission times or even moving house. Wearing a mask when cycling through the middle of heavy traffic affords some protection (see page 114 for further information on these masks).

Avoid cigarette smoke

One of the biggest sources of pollution in homes and offices is smoking. Cigarette smoke is a potent brew of toxic chemicals, including cyanide and ammonia – and the well-known, and terrible, diseases linked to smoking range from lung cancer to emphysema. Apart from hanging in the air, cigarette smoke will also soak into your clothes and furnishings and lurk there for days, slowly seeping back into the atmosphere.

Obviously, if you're smoking and you value your health – and you wouldn't be reading this book if you didn't – you need to quit. Once you've done that, you'll need to make your home a no-smoking area, and create a fuss at work if smoking is still allowed there. Let visitors to your house know when they arrive that as much as you like them, you have difficulty with their smoking indoors. If really pushed, even put up a small sign. Going out can be a problem, but an increasing number of restaurants and bars are adopting no-smoking policies, so seek them out.

Scent danger

Many household products directly or indirectly feed chemicals into the air or get into your body by other routes. Some of the worst offenders are fairly pointless products that we can do without, but others are everyday staples. You can buy 'holistic' alternatives to pretty well all of them, sometimes even from your local supermarket, but I won't pretend this isn't sometimes a hassle. Once again, how far you go to root out problem products from your home depends on how sensitive you are and how badly they affect you.

As far as possible, don't use ...   Products that might give off a vapour (in technical language – anything 'volatile') or that has a scent. When you can smell something it means that receptors in your nose are picking up tiny packets of chemicals given off by that product, so that anything with a scent is by definition giving off a chemical vapour. Often the stronger something smells, the more likely it is to trigger a sensitivity reaction. Also avoid products with chemicals that might get onto your skin or into your mouth.

A list of things to avoid includes:

- Scented toiletries of all sorts, including soap, powder, perfume, shampoo, aftershave, moisturiser, roll-on or stick deodorants/antiperspirants, bubble bath, bath salts and talcum power. Toothpastes (especially gels) typically contain a lot of additives (such as preservatives, artificial sweeteners like aspartame and saccharine, and detergents), which can trigger reactions. Good alternatives that work are those based on sodium bicarbonate – you can find these products in health food stores

- All aerosols or sprays, including air fresheners, fly spray or spray deodorant/anti-perspirant

- Scented or synthetic cleaning materials, including bathroom, kitchen, window and oven cleaners

- Highly scented biological washing powders; conditioners and fabric softeners

- Furniture/carpet cleaners/fresheners, such as spray-on or powder-and-vacuum products, perfumed vacuum cleaner bags

- Polish (floor, furniture and so on), varnish, glue (including that on the backs of stamps/envelopes), vinyl paint. Be sure to ventilate adequately rooms in which you are using these products.

The list above includes a lot of products that might seem indispensable to modern life, but don't despair – it is possible to clean your home, clothes and self without exposing your system to loads of toxic substances. Two of the key replacement substances are borax and bicarbonate of soda, old-fashioned, simple cleaning agents that very rarely trigger reactions.

Do use . . . The substances and products that follow are effective for cleaning your house, and you, without causing any health problems:

- Unscented vegetable soap for the bath, sink and shower, and plain soap shampoo from health food shops (mainstream commercial varieties of 'pure' or 'natural'/herbal soap may still contain additives)

- 'Homeopathic' or herbal varieties of toothpaste, or, for a really hypoallergenic mouthwash, try mixing two parts bicarbonate of soda with one part sea salt

- Borax or bicarbonate of soda for cleaning floors and kitchen and bathroom surfaces

- Bicarbonate of soda instead of oven cleaner. Hot fat and bicarbonate of soda react together to form a crude soap. By smearing bicarbonate of soda over the inside of your oven you can do away with the need for toxic oven cleaners – splashes of grease will turn to soap, which can be easily washed away. Even better, some ovens and range cookers like Agas almost never need to be cleaned!

- Washing soda for toilets and drains

- Plain laundry washing powders or, for the really sensitive, pure soap or bicarbonate of soda

- Beeswax to polish floors

- An air filter with an activated charcoal filter to 'scrub' the air clean in your home. You could also fit water filters or purifiers to your water supply or to individual taps to ensure a cleaner water supply. (One of my patients, Emma, suffered terrible itching when she showered – until she fitted a special shower head to remove irritating chemicals.)

Like my mother and grandmother, I use all these things – and they do work.

The cleaning product 'exclusion diet'   If you're looking to cut down on your domestic chemical exposure because you suspect that something is triggering specific symptoms of chemical sensitivity, such as headaches or fatigue, but don't want to give up all your household products at once, you could try a sort of 'exclusion diet'. As with food, this involves cutting out as many potential triggers as possible and then gradually reintroducing them.

First gather up all the suspect products described above and pack them away in a garage or outhouse if possible, or an attic if not. Air the house as much as possible to flush out lingering vapours. If your symptoms improve after two to three weeks, you can move on to the next stage. If not, it either means that you need to be even more ruthless in your banishment of potential trigger products, or that your symptoms are caused by an outside source (something at work or more general pollution).

Assuming that your symptoms do improve, reintroduce the products you miss most, one at a time. Don't start off by spraying them all over the house – try sniffing the product first, then using it in one room only, monitoring your reactions the whole time. Wait a week before reintroducing the next one.

The office or workplace is an environment you have less control over, but office cleaners and janitors often use very strong cleaning chemicals packed full of solvents, chlorine, ammonia and phenol. Not only are these products usually stronger than domestic versions, they are often supplied in concentrated form in large quantities for the cleaner to dilute, which may not get done properly. If you suspect that the office environment is making you feel ill, try and get your office manager to review the products used and consider hypoallergenic substitutes. One patient, Marie, suffered headaches at work but not at home. We realised the office photocopier was the trigger as she was clearly sensitive to the VOCs released by the machine. Once the copier was moved to another room, Marie's headaches cleared up.

BUILT-IN DANGERS

Structural sources of chemical pollution can include all sorts of furniture and fittings. The worst offenders tend to be particle board (found in walls, floors and furniture) and new carpets, but practically any synthetic or treated materials can cause problems or add to your toxic load. Here are a few tips to help you avoid some of the worst problems:

- Anti-mite strategies for floor coverings tend to be healthier – including wooden, cork or tiled floors, or linoleum (made from linseed oil, sawdust and sailcloth). However, many wood products are treated before installation. You can either try sticking to hardwoods, which need minimal treatment but are expensive and may not be ecologically friendly, or be prepared to let a new floor air out for some time. Try to avoid synthetic varnishes and polishes – stick to wax or linseed oil.

- Avoid using particle boards in woodwork or furniture.

- If you are buying a carpet or other material, make sure you smell it first. The stronger the smell, the more problems it's likely to cause. A handy tip is to cut off a square of material and put it in a jar with the lid closed. Leave it in a warm place for a few days and then smell it, before deciding whether or not to buy it.

- If you already have a carpet and it smells, improve the ventilation in the room and think about getting it steam cleaned. An air filter with an activated charcoal filter might come in useful. Alternatively, try hanging the carpet to air in the garage for a while.

- Avoid synthetic fabrics on your furnishings – use cotton, linen or hemp instead.

- Decorating can introduce loads of toxic chemicals into your home all at once. Decorate in the summer months when paint, for instance, will dry quickly, and ensure your house is well ventilated. Think about staying somewhere else until it's aired out. Don't use vinyl paints.

Shop around for less polluting products, such as water-based varnish or solvent-free paints.

- As I have said, gas cookers and boilers give off a lot of toxic fumes. The simplest way to avoid such problems is to switch to electric heating and cooking or have your boiler away from the main living area in a ventilated space. If this isn't practical, make sure your gas appliances are well maintained and vented, and get an expert in at least annually to measure emissions. The best place for a gas boiler is in an outhouse, or failing that in a separate and very well-ventilated room. If you suspect that a gas appliance may still be causing you problems, check before undertaking major alterations. Turn off the gas supply for at least ten days and monitor your symptoms.

Avoid toxic metals

While some metallic elements – such as zinc, copper and iron – are important micronutrients (see Chapter 5), metals can be dangerous to your health, especially if they're allowed to build up in your body. Particular problem metals include lead, mercury, cadmium and aluminium. These substances do not have to be present in the body at clinically toxic levels to be damaging your system. What's known as sub-acute poisoning has been linked to all sorts of health problems – sub-acute lead poisoning, for instance, may cause learning and behavioural problems, kidney disease, stillbirth, and chronic fatigue. You can reduce your risk of exposure in a number of ways:

- Don't smoke, and try to avoid other people's smoke and ash. Cigarette ash, which makes up part of the smoke, is rich in toxic metals.

- Avoid aluminium and unlined copper cooking utensils.

- Get your plumbing system checked to make sure it isn't contaminated or in disrepair. Lead leaches into the water from lead pipes which may be in your home or from the mains supply.

- If you buy fruit or veg from stalls outside shops next to busy roads make sure you wash it very thoroughly, or peel it – it can be contaminated with lead from air pollution.

- Take your shoes off when you come in to the house, and vacuum frequently – we all bring contaminants and pollutants into the house with us on our shoes, via particulate matter that has settled on the ground.

- Think about wearing a mask if you cycle or walk near heavy traffic. Good-quality masks have an activated charcoal filter, a sooty substance with billions of tiny holes that soak up and lock away toxins. Eventually the filter will fill up and the mask will have to be replaced.

- Be careful with lead models and toys (such as toy soldiers or figurines), and don't give them to children.

- If you have a hobby, such as ceramics, you may be at risk of exposure to heavy metals. Check with the Health and Safety Executive about every material you use. Treat yourself with the same care that is expected of an employer towards an employee.

- There is growing evidence of the possible danger of permanent chemical hair dyes – especially darker colours. Long-term exposure may be linked with lymphoma – a form of cancer affecting glands. If you dye your hair, consider semi-permanent dyes, and follow health recommendations as they emerge.

PART **3**

Physical Health

CHAPTER 9

DIY body screening

W e've taken a long, in-depth look at biochemical health and the factors that influence it, particularly nutrition and our home and work environments. Now, harking back to our triangle of health, it's time to look at the physical corner – the obvious, visible, palpable aspect of our wellbeing.

Start by thinking back to your last GP consultation. Were you hurried in and out with just enough time to mention your symptoms and receive a prescription? Or was your visit part of an integrated plan for managing and maintaining your health, during which you felt that your doctor discussed your concerns and options, based on your ongoing monitoring of your health?

Perhaps the second scenario sounds a bit far-fetched, but it shouldn't – for I hope this is how my own patients recall their consultations with me.

In order to look after your physical wellbeing, you have to be fairly vigilant about it, knowing when to see your doctor and what to ask him or her so that you get the best out of your doctor–patient partnership.

TAKE CHARGE OF YOUR HEALTH

1. **Know your body**. Keeping track of what's normal for your body and what is not will give you the information you need to take a problem to your GP.

---

2. **Do your homework**. If you notice anything new or different, keep a short diary of symptoms, or jot down dates that will help keep track of a problem. Before your appointment, condense your notes down to the main points.

3. **Ask the right questions**. In the heat of the moment during a medical consultation, a short list of questions will keep you on track, and you're less likely to come away thinking you're still none the wiser. If you don't understand something, ask your doctor to explain it another way, or ask if he or she can suggest a book or leaflet on the subject. And never be afraid to ask a 'silly question' – there aren't any, when it comes to your health. Moreover, if needing to know something is making you anxious, it's very important to set your mind at rest.

4. **Be assertive, not aggressive**. You may have been biting your nails about the consultation. But GPs can get anxious too. A lot of their professional magazines now offer advice on 'coping with the well-informed and demanding patient'. Just knowing this may give you a sense of power. But the rapport between you will be better if you can avoid being bullish.

5. **Help your doctor out**. Say: 'I have three questions,' so he or she knows what's coming. And, even if you've read up about your symptoms and have a pretty good idea of what they could be, try not to bombard your doc with a textbook diagnosis. You may end up learning nothing new if you come across as knowing it all already, and the consultation may then become a waste of effort. If you have cuttings or information from the internet, show him or her – then he or she can advise you or make further enquiries on your behalf.

The next few chapters are aimed at showing you how to monitor your own physical health. I'll tell you some of the things that I look out for in my patients, and how you can look out for them yourself. I'll tell you a bit about what they might mean, so if you notice any worrying symptoms yourself, you'll be able to go to the doctor armed with some relevant questions.

As well as the obvious symptoms of physical health, we'll also look at factors that can affect your health such as poor posture or lack of exercise, and I'll give you some useful tips for exercises that you can use to remedy problems in these areas.

And finally, Part 3 also discusses your role as a patient: the health tests you can request, and your relationship with your family doctor. Are you getting the most out of the options available to you?

This section covers topics you might not ordinarily think of as being anything to do with physical health, but by this time you probably know that I believe that all aspects of our lives are interrelated. My philosophy is that the more you look after each and every aspect of your life, the more in-tune and healthy you'll be.

CHAPTER 10

Signs and symptoms

When I'm assessing a patient, complex lab-based tests come second to the assessment I can make with my own eyes and hands. If you know what to look for, you can tell a great deal about a person's reserves of health, lifestyle, likely family history and their predisposition to certain conditions, simply by listening to their story and examining their appearance in detail.

The key to such an assessment is years of training and experience, and unfortunately that's something I can't get across in a book. However, in these chapters I *can* give you direction for a preliminary self-assessment that you can do at home just by looking in the mirror. Remember that a self-assessment should only be a first step – if you suspect you have any symptoms of a serious condition, you must always check with your doctor, and you shouldn't start or alter treatments without expert advice.

■ Assessing your appearance and symptoms

- Is your hair greasy, dry, unmanageable or prematurely grey?

- Is your scalp itchy or flaky?

- Is your face puffy or flaccid?

- Do you have flaky or greasy skin on your forehead, cheeks or on either side of your nose?

- Is your skin extremely oily or dry?

- Do you suffer from excess facial or body hair?

- Do you suffer from acne?

- Do you have premature wrinkles?

- Do you have dark circles under your eyes?

- Are your eyes bloodshot or bulging?

- Do you suffer from frequent cold sores or cracks at the corners of your mouth?

- Do you have bleeding or retracted gums?

- Is your tongue furry, dry or cracked? Has it become red and sore?

- Do you suffer from recurrent mouth ulcers?

- Do you have a swollen neck or swollen glands?

- Do you have white spots on your nails?

- Does your urine have any of the following characteristics? Cloudy, frothy, dark or strangely coloured; bloody; offensive smell; discomfort, burning or stinging on urination.

- For men, does your urine come out in a strong, steady stream with a sharp cut-off, or is the flow weaker and prolonged?

What can you tell from looking in the mirror?

The evidence of your skin, hair, eyes and body is a guide to your physical health. The appearance of your features reflects what and how much you eat, drink and smoke, your physical and social environment including stress levels and sleep patterns and your physiological/ 'real' (as opposed to your chronological) age. They can provide clues to any illness that might be affecting you, even before it becomes clinically apparent, and possibly even to diseases that may affect you in the future.

■ Is your hair greasy, dry, unmanageable or prematurely grey?

Dry or unmanageable hair can be a warning sign of a poorly functioning thyroid gland, other hormone disturbances, or a poor diet. Greasy hair may just be normal for you, but may also be a sign of hormonal imbalance or, if you're a woman, of hormonal fluctuations during your menstrual cycle. Premature greying – for example in your twenties – is sometimes hereditary, but can also be a sign of nutritional deficiency, such as protein or iron deficiency. A condition called pernicious anaemia, which causes failure of vitamin B12 absorption, may also be characterised by early greying.

■ Is your scalp itchy or flaky?

An itchy or flaky scalp may indicate eczema, either local, caused by direct contact with an irritant, or systemic (also known as atopic), where contact with an allergen triggers an allergic response all through the body. It can also be a sign of psoriasis or infestation with lice (typically in schoolchildren). Dandruff can be a warning sign of yeast infection or seborrhoeic dermatitis.

SIX REASONS FOR AN ITCHY SCALP

1. **Dandruff** Somewhat similar to seborrhoeic dermatitis, dandruff is caused by an overgrowth of scalp yeasts, especially when you're under stress or your hormones are out of kilter. Calm down the yeast activity with a treatment containing tea tree oil or mahonia. Both are widely available from chemists and health food stores.

2. **Contact dermatitis** The scalp can develop this allergic reaction and skin

---

irritations to chemicals in shampoos, conditioners and hair dye. Change hair products every couple of months or so, always rinse thoroughly in cool or tepid water, and avoid chemical products as far as possible.

3. **Scalp psoriasis** This is most likely if you are already prone to patches of psoriasis elsewhere on your body. Psoriasis is a condition in which skin cells multiply too fast, creating patches of raised, reddened skin covered with adherent scales. To remove the scaly patches, use a coal tar shampoo which your GP can prescribe. I see many patients with psoriasis and find it a particularly rewarding condition to manage.

4. **Neurodermatitis** Neurodermatitis characteristically occurs on the nape of the neck, and continual scratching causes the area of skin to become thickened, reddened and itchy. This condition often flares up during periods of particular anxiety or in people suffering from long-term anxiety. Having excluded any other scalp condition, the best way to treat it is to break the itch and scratch cycle. Anxiety reduction techniques and relaxation exercises can also help.

5. **Tinea** A ringworm-type fungal infection, tinea affects children's scalps more than adults' – and usually involves some hair loss, too, in a characteristic 'ring' pattern. You should see your GP, who will take skin scrapings to confirm a suspected diagnosis. Do not delay, as this is infectious.

6. **Head lice** Ironically, head lice love clean hair. Here's how you tackle them. Wash hair and then apply conditioner. Careful combing with a fine-toothed 'nit' comb can help the insects and eggs slide out and be removed. Very persistent cases may require pesticide treatment from your doctor or pharmacy, but this should be avoided if at all possible. Again, head lice spread like wildfire, so act promptly.

■ Is your face puffy or flaccid?

A puffy or flaccid face is usually a sign of either illness or overindulgence – too many late nights, too much drinking and smoking, and too little quality food. It may also be a sign of an underactive thyroid gland, and sometimes of kidney disorder, so you should discuss these possibilities with your doctor.

■ What's the skin like on your forehead, cheeks or on either side of your nose?

Flaking and/or greasiness of the forehead, the sides of the nose and the cheeks, together with dandruff, can be a sign of seborrhoeic eczema – an oily, yeasty eczema. Sometimes seborrhoeic eczema is linked to food intolerance.

ALL TOGETHER NOW: OILY SKIN, ACNE, EXCESS HAIR

Androgens such as testosterone can cause more than oily skin. They may also be the culprit behind acne and excess body and facial hair. These conditions may also indicate a disorder of the ovaries or adrenal glands, although acne is, of course, 'normal' round puberty. Women with these conditions should be checked for polycystic ovarian syndrome and may have irregular periods.

■ Is your skin oily or dry?

Extreme dryness can indicate hormonal imbalance, for example an underactive thyroid (thyroid dysfunction is surprisingly widespread). It may also indicate a lack of oils and foods rich in essential fatty acids in your diet. Some people do tend towards oilier skin, as do adolescents. However, if it has only recently appeared, it may indicate a hormone imbalance – maybe an increase in androgen (male type) hormones. This should be checked out by blood tests for hormone levels. Your doctor may order blood tests for hormone levels, especially if there are other symptoms such as (for a woman) irregular periods or excess facial hair.

◼ Do you suffer from excess hair?

Hirsuitism – excessive facial or body hair – may simply reflect your constitutional type or heredity. But, if it doesn't seem to be a family trait, it could be a sign of a hormone problem such as polycystic ovarian syndrome (which, untreated, leaves some women subfertile and may put you at increased risk of heart disease and diabetes). There's also a chance that your increased hair growth could be due to an ovarian or adrenal tumour, so book in with a doctor for hormone level tests straight away to find the underlying cause before you even think about expensive hair removal treatments. If it's nothing serious but you're finding the hair difficult to deal with, be aware that electrolysis or laser treatment is available free of charge on the NHS in some parts of the UK. If you live outside the UK, it's worth asking your doctor if this is the case where you live.

◼ Do you have acne?

Acne can also be linked to conditions influencing hormone levels. However, it's often a sign of poor dietary habits and a generally unhealthy lifestyle.

◼ Are you prematurely wrinkled?

Wrinkles and other signs of apparently premature ageing may show that your physiological age is outstripping your chronological age – a phenomenon discussed in Chapter 20. If you're wrinkled beyond your years, you may well be overexposing yourself to harmful UV rays in sunlight, smoking, drinking too much and failing to get enough vitamins, essential fatty acids and other micronutrients from your diet.

◼ Do you have dark circles under your eyes?

Dark circles under the eyes are caused by seepage of fluid from the tiny capillaries around the eyes – a kind of 'mini-bruising'. They can be linked to allergies, but are more commonly the result of insufficient/disrupted sleep (see Chapter 18), smoking and heavy drinking – all the elements of an unhealthy lifestyle.

'I'VE GOT BAGS UNDER MY EYES!'

Sue, a secretary in her thirties, came to see me about unsightly bags that had been developing under her eyes. They'd been bad for some time but at first she had simply put it down to a period of overwork. Now she was worried she'd never get rid of them, and that they were making her look old. On top of that, her long-standing hay fever seemed to be getting worse, with symptoms afflicting her all year round instead of just during the summer.

Dark circles under the eyes can be a symptom of allergy, so it seemed likely that the bags and the allergy were closely linked and getting worse due to a common factor. We discussed Sue's lifestyle and it quickly became apparent that she was burning the candle at both ends – going out drinking and partying most nights of the week and getting by with too few hours of sleep. I pointed out that not only was this almost certainly taking its toll on her skin, but the smoky environments, unhealthy diet and lack of sleep were also likely to be aggravating her allergy.

Obviously Sue wasn't going to transform from 'good-time girl' to nun overnight, but we agreed on a plan to improve her diet, increase the amount of sleep she was allowing herself and try to keep away from cigarette smoke. Her allergic symptoms improved somewhat, and so did the bags under her eyes. Perhaps more importantly, Sue now knows what she needs to do to improve her health and appearance – everything else is up to her!

■ Are your eyes bloodshot or bulging?

Bulging eyes can be a sign of conditions such as an overactive thyroid gland and should be reported immediately. Bloodshot or reddened eyes can be the result of eye strain (staring at a screen or page for long periods without blinking enough dries out the eyes), lack of sleep, allergy or infection. Rheumatic disorders may also affect the eyes, causing inflammation and redness.

▪ Are you plagued by cold sores or cracks at the corners of your mouth?

Cold sores are caused by a variety of the herpes virus that many people carry. Most of the time it lies dormant, but if your immune system is weakened or overtaxed the virus can reactivate and cause a cold sore. If you get a lot of them, it's a strong indicator that your reserves of health are overstretched and your immune system isn't working at full throttle.

Cracks in the corner of the mouth are known as angular stomatitis, a condition that can be a warning sign of iron or vitamin B deficiency, especially in those not eating a nutritionally sound diet, the anaemic or the elderly.

▪ How healthy are your gums?

Bleeding gums are usually a symptom of gingivitis – inflammation of the gums around the teeth due to a build-up of plaque and bacterial infection. But they can occasionally be a serious symptom (for example, a blood disorder, or even scurvy, caused by vitamin C deficiency – though this is thankfully extremely rare these days). See your dentist or doctor straight away for assessment. Retracted gums can be a sign of ageing, overbrushing or brushing too hard, smoking or poor nutrition.

▪ What's the state of your tongue like?

A furry tongue is often a sign of poor oral hygiene (many people don't realise that you're supposed to brush your tongue as well as your teeth). A dry tongue can be a symptom of auto-immune problems. A sore, red tongue may indicate iron or vitamin B deficiency. White patches on a sore tongue may be a sign of a yeast infection (such as thrush, caused by *Candida albicans*). Any mouth or tongue problem that continues for several weeks must be seen by a doctor, as oral cancers are sadly very common and early diagnosis is essential.

■ Do you have recurrent mouth ulcers?

Recurrent mouth ulcers may simply mean that you need some of your teeth filed down slightly, or that your dentures don't fit properly. But an ulcer that recurs or does not heal over three weeks or so could be a sign of mouth cancer or rarer conditions such as Behcet's disease – see a doctor straight away.

■ Do you have a swollen neck or swollen glands?

The thyroid gland sits in the centre of the neck over the Adam's apple, and can swell – a condition known as goitre. Nodules may also occur in the gland, causing swelling. Swollen glands can also be caused by a variety of diseases. Some are mild and self-limiting, like a sore throat caused by a virus. Others may be more serious and require urgent investigations – for example, some cancers or TB.

■ Do you have white spots on your nails?

White spots on the nails can be a sign of zinc deficiency, but they can also be caused by trauma to the nails, such as a knock, so you may be prone to these marks if you do a lot of typing or manual work. If zinc deficiency is to blame your nails should improve within a few months of adding more zinc-rich foods (such as oatmeal, nuts, oysters or eggs) to your diet, or starting a course of zinc supplementation if this has been advised. This is actually one of the most common deficiencies I see, and zinc is crucial to your health. A deficiency can result in weakened immunity, and may be a factor in skin problems, slow wound healing, psychiatric problems, impotence, infertility and low libido, dandruff, impaired taste and smell, reduced appetite . . . in fact, this list alone is impressive enough to convince most people to take good nutrition seriously!

■ Do you have healthy urination?

Your kidneys actively filter your blood to remove excess water and a variety of impurities, waste products and toxins – the end result is urine. Urine can be assessed at a doctor's surgery with stick testing, where a plastic stick coated with reagents is dipped into a urine sample to test for pH, the presence of blood (red and white cells) and levels of glucose, protein, nitrite or bilirubin (a blood breakdown product).

Some signs of ill health, however, may be indicated simply by looking at a sample of urine. Warning signs to look out for include cloudy or frothy urine, visible debris in the urine, dark or strangely coloured urine, blood, or an offensive or unusual odour. Discomfort, burning or stinging on urination give further clues. Symptoms like this are suggestive of a urinary tract infection (UTI) or sexually transmitted infection (STI). (Do not ignore this – see your doctor or clinic, and if an STI is diagnosed tell your partner who should also attend for screening and treatment.) If your urine is often quite concentrated, you're probably not drinking enough water. A well-hydrated person will have almost colourless urine. Abnormal findings in urine may also indicate diabetes (the presence of glucose) or kidney disease (the presence of protein). Protein may cause a frothy appearance.

■ If you're a man, do you urinate in a strong, steady stream with a sharp cut-off?

The way in which urine comes out can be a good indicator of prostate health. A strong, steady stream with a sharp cut-off is healthy. Hesitancy (reluctance of urine to emerge), weak flow and dribbling at the end of urination are suggestive of prostate problems, particularly in older men. Ask your doctor about prostate screening.

Socrates's philosophic cornerstone – 'Know thyself' – doesn't just apply to the inner self. It's also wise to get to know your own body. That thorough look in the mirror is key to good health. Understanding when something may be wrong, because it's not normal *for you*, will enable you to get the help you need. For more about the many specialist screening tests available, see Chapter 14.

CHAPTER 11

Gut reaction

In Part 2, you examined what you were eating, and how you were eating it. But as I indicated at that point, it is just as important to turn detective and examine what you are producing as a result of your diet. I encourage all my patients to look at what they have left in the toilet bowl, and to discuss the frequency and pattern to their bowel movements. In this busy, busy world, where most of us have too little time for anything that is not absolutely essential, it is easy to get into the habit of ignoring the natural urge to open the bowel. This, especially when combined with a poor-quality diet, can result in a range of symptoms including headaches, lethargy and skin complaints as well as the gut reactions, such as vague abdominal pains, you would naturally expect. Think about your answers to the questions below. In the rest of the chapter we'll be looking at some common gut problems and how to deal with them.

■ The state of your bowels

- Are your bowel movements regularly characterised by any of the following features? Unformed or liquid stool; smelly, very dark or very light-coloured stool; large amounts of gas; offensive-smelling gas; feeling of incomplete emptying; anal itchiness; sudden urgency; forcing; leaving marks on the toilet bowl; requiring a lot of toilet paper.

- Do you have blood or slime in your stool or on your toilet paper?

- Have your bowel habits or the frequency of your movements changed?

- Do you have four or more of the following symptoms? Fatigue or low energy levels; poor concentration; dry skin/eczema; susceptibility to thrush infection; excessive wind; bloating; feeling tired after meals; anal itchiness.

■ How are your bowel movements?

When I qualified as a doctor, I attended a lecture given by a medical colleague of the highly respected Denis Burkitt. He had worked in Africa with a local community and had found that the usual gut disorders treated in Western countries were rarely a problem for the indigenous peoples. Bowel cancers, haemorrhoids, gallstones, diverticular disease and appendicitis were a rarity. Yet these are the core of a Western general surgeon's daily workload. Burkitt studied the stools of the local people for clues about their gut health and found that it was mostly soft with bits of root vegetables and seeds in it. As we young doctors sat and watched a succession of delightful slides showing different types of poo, he explained that this diet – one we in the West had given up quite a while ago – was responsible for the almost complete lack of gastroenterological complications in these people. It was Denis Burkitt's work that introduced the medical world to the importance of a high-fibre diet and highlighted the perils of the high-protein, high-sugar and refined carbohydrate diet of the West.

'BUT MY DIET'S NORMAL, ISN'T IT?'

James was referred to me by a surgeon. For 10 years, from the age of 17, he had been going to the loo up to 14 times a day, and was troubled by embarrassing wind and bloating. He was eating red meat six times a week and white meat three times a week. He ate no breakfast, and lunch was a sandwich while walking or working if he wasn't out on a work lunch (for a steak). Dinner was erratic, and he hardly ever ate fruit or vegetables. He never ate fish (fish and veg made him hungry for a Big Mac!), but had thick white bread three or four times a day. When a doctor suspects gut dysbiosis, as I did with James, it is possible to order a blood test to measure gut fermentation, through the levels of ethanol (alcohol) that the gut produces in response to a dose of sugar. This is not often necessary, but is an elegant way to demonstrate the fermentation process and alcohol production within the gut.

When I ran this test on James, it transpired he was producing 146 units of ethanol, compared to the 'normal' level one would expect of up to just 22 units! His was a classic case of gut dysbiosis. Like so many patients, James hoped I would give him a one-off fix. Of course I couldn't, but he was happy to accept my advice that he should go on a new regime and make fundamental changes to the way he shopped, cooked and ate – and is now following my gut dysbiosis programme (see below). But bear in mind that it is vital not to manage bowel disorders yourself. Symptoms such as James's must be medically investigated to ensure there is no underlying pathology such as inflammatory bowel disease or polyps.

So how should a healthy stool look? It should be sausage-shaped, passed in one piece and have a smooth surface. As the anal ring closes after evacuating, one end of the soft but formed stool will have a slightly pointed end. It sinks in water because it is not loaded with gas, and has only a slight characteristic odour. It shouldn't be too strong smelling, as this may be a sign of intestinal fermentation.

A healthy intestine evacuates the stool cleanly, which is why any noticeable soiling of the anal region is an indication of disturbed digestion. In other words, if you have to use a lot of toilet paper or you're leaving marks on the bowl, your digestive system isn't functioning properly.

In contrast to the healthy stool, the unhealthy bowel movement is either very hard (in the case of constipation), unformed or liquid, smelly, very dark or very light coloured, and accompanied by large amounts of gas, or offensive smelling gas. A sensation of incomplete emptying of the bowels, anal itchiness, sudden urgency or forcing are also bad signs.

◼ Is there blood or slime evident?

Blood in the stool or on the paper after wiping means that your gastro-intestinal tract is bleeding. This may have a benign cause such as haemor-rhoids or it could be a symptom of something serious like cancer. See a doctor immediately, even if you've already been diagnosed with haemor-rhoids – serious and simple disorders can coexist. Mucus or slime that is present with the stool can be a symptom of irritable bowel syndrome (IBS), intestinal infection, diverticulosis, inflammatory bowel disease or a tumour.

◼ Have your bowel habits changed?

The regularity of your bowel movements is more important than the frequency. A *change* in the frequency of bowel movements or other aspects of bowel habit (such as blood, slime or loose, frequent stool) can be a symptom of digestive problems or a warning sign for cancer, particularly in older people. Report any change to your doctor, who will examine you and consider referral for investigations, which may include:

- Colonoscopy (using fibre optics, a full internal inspection of the colon)

- A barium enema (an X-ray imaging technique for bowel inspection).

HOW ARE YOUR MOVEMENTS?

- Type 1: Separate hard lumps, like nuts or goat droppings

- Type 2: Sausage-shaped, but lumpy like goat droppings pushed together

- Type 3: Like a sausage, smooth and soft

- Type 4: Soft blobs with clear-cut edges (passed easily), may stick to toilet bowl

- Type 5: Fluffy pieces with ragged edges, a mushy stool, may float

- Type 6: Watery, no solid pieces; entirely liquid

Remember, stools should be passed as a process of relaxation, giving a sense of complete emptying. Incomplete emptying is very common and indicates the need for dietary adjustment.

WHAT IT SAYS ABOUT YOU:

- Type 3: Congratulations! You have perfectly normal bowel movements. Ideally you should be having this kind of bowel movement once a day, or maybe twice.

- Types 1 & 2: Are abnormally hard and solid, indicating constipation, and result from a slow bowel transit time. These seem over the long term to be linked with an increased risk of diverticular disease and piles.

- Type 4: Is poorly formed, fat, sticky, soft and verging on abnormal.

- Type 5 & 6: Are abnormally loose, indicating diarrhoea. You and your doctor should seek the underlying cause if this persists, especially if there has been a change in bowel habits or appearance.

■ Do you suffer from symptoms of gut dysbiosis?

Gut dysbiosis affects the delicately balanced ecosystem that exists in the human gut. Normally, over 500 species of bacteria coexist in your lower intestines, feeding off partially digested food and each other, and producing a range of important biochemicals upon which your own system depends. Although the numbers of each species fluctuate, in the healthy or 'eubiotic' gut there is an overall balance.

If this balance is disrupted, with some species of bacteria proliferating at the expense of others, your system becomes 'dysbiotic', which can lead to a variety of symptoms. Individually the symptoms could indicate any one of dozens of causes, but there is a characteristic pattern, or constellation, of symptoms that indicates dysbiosis.

The central features of the dysbiotic constellation are gut problems such as excessive wind, bloating and feeling tired after meals. Women may be susceptible to vaginal thrush infection. Some people suffer fatigue and low energy. If these symptoms sound familiar, check your food diary. Patients who develop dysbiosis often eat erratically, skipping meals and consuming lots of sugars, either refined or from natural sources such as fruit, and eating lots of fermented foods such as Marmite, tea, alcohol, blue cheese or soy sauce.

What can you do if you think you might be suffering from dysbiosis? I would consider ordering a test called a gut fermentation profile. However, a simple diagnostic step you can take yourself is to cut out the foods mentioned above and follow some of the dietary tips discussed below. Improvement of symptoms after following an anti-dysbiosis diet (usually for at least three weeks) is the best confirmation that you had dysbiosis in the first place.

'HAVE I GOT GUT DYSBIOSIS?'

Mark, a fortysomething TV producer, had come to see me complaining of eczema, anal itchiness and general fatigue. His GP had treated some of his symptoms with steroid antifungal creams but had had little success in achieving sustained improvement or in identifying the underlying causes. Mark had also sought help from several alternative therapists, but had been given treatments and dietary advice that had severely limited the range of foods he was 'allowed'. This had had little or no effect. Worse, he had suffered a delay in getting effective treatment. He was a shadow of his former self, had lost a lot of weight and was depressed about his illness and unable to keep up with his usual frantic schedule.

Such a diverse constellation of symptoms led me to suspect dysbiosis, but it's absolutely vital to consider the full range of possible diagnoses and rule out the more serious ones first, so I made sure to undertake a full range of conventional screenings. A gut fermentation profile test revealed that he did indeed have fungal-type gut dysbiosis, and by simply altering his diet and making recommendations to encourage the growth of healthy gut flora and restore overall balance to his gut, Mark's symptoms were relieved. Within a month or so he was back to his usual self and cheered up immensely.

Treating gut dysbiosis

The management of poor bowel habit and dysbiosis takes most patients right back to basics. They often have to retrain their bowel – learning the kind of toilet training habits that would have come naturally to them as very young children. They also need to spring-clean their diet (I use the bowel cleansing programme and low-sugar, low-yeast diet, below) and rebalance the flora of their gut with probiotic foods and, sometimes, supplements of healthy probiotic bacteria.

Bowel retraining Make a point of going to the toilet after breakfast every morning. If you tend not to open your bowels easily, sit with your feet on a low footstool to raise your knees and improve your centre of gravity to stimulate the bowel to start moving its contents in the right direction. Any straining is absolutely forbidden. Instead, to get things moving, try sipping a glass of water, or massaging your tummy in a clockwise direction (see below).

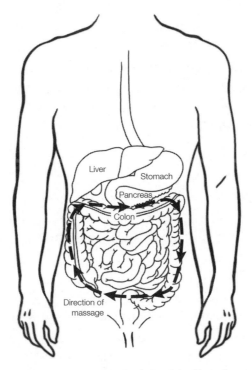

Massage your stomach in this direction

Bowel cleansing programme For two to three days maximum, eat only from the following list.

- **Fruit juices** diluted by half with bottled water. Avoid juices made from concentrates. Try apple, pear, papaya, fresh orange and black cherry juices.

- **Vegetable juices** diluted by a third with bottled water. Combine one from each of the following groups: a) Apple or carrot juice (4oz/110g) b) Dark green lettuce, celery or cucumber juice (4–6oz/110–170g) c) Parsley, beetroot, red cabbage, spinach (1–2oz/30–60g).

If doing this amount of juicing is difficult for you, or you don't have access to a juicer, buy bottled organic vegetable juices from health food shops.

- **Mineral-rich Bieler broth** (two bowls a day). To make, chop up and steam two medium courgettes, 4oz (110g) green beans and two stalks of celery. Place them in a blender with a handful of chopped parsley or coriander and enough of the water used for steaming to make two to three bowls.

- **Alkaline broth** (2–3 bowls per day). To make, use a stainless steel saucepan. Fill with 1.5 litres of water, add two washed, chopped but unpeeled potatoes, 1 cup of chopped carrots, 1 cup of diced celery and 1 cup of another root vegetable, such as swede, chopped. Add cayenne, basil, oregano and other desired seasonings. Cover and cook on a low heat until the vegetables are very soft. Allow to cool for another half an hour and strain, drinking only the broth.

- **Herb teas,** but no coffee, black tea or any other caffeinated drink.

When following a semi-fast like this, you must rest, limit yourself to 'home activities' and take only gentle exercise such as walking. Those with an existing medical condition must not follow dietary restrictions without medical approval and supervision.

The anti-dysbiosis diet Restoring the balance of your gut flora means you need to pay careful attention to your diet for at least several weeks. Below are lists of what to eat and drink, to encourage the return of healthy bacteria and reduce the overgrowth of harmful bacteria and yeasts.

The diet is mixed and varied, and meat and fish may be eaten. It doesn't exclude any major food groups. Vary your diet as much as possible and make a real effort to find and eat foods you don't usually have. Many people rarely touch pulses and millet, for example.

Here are the elements of the diet:

- **Vegetables.** Eat fresh organic vegetables, raw, steamed, boiled or stir-fried with a little oil. Include plenty of garlic, which has anti-fungal properties: up to two cloves of cooked garlic a day is optimal, along with raw garlic in salad or vegetable dressings.

- **Meat and fish.** Eat lean, organic meat and fish.

- **Grains.** Eat organic whole grains – whole wheat, oats, barley, rye, millet, buckwheat, maize, brown rice and wholemeal pasta. Don't eat ordinary bread made with yeast. Substitute unleavened bread (scones, chapattis, pita bread, soda bread, crackers or rice cakes).

- **Fruit.** Eat a maximum of two pieces of lower-sugar fruit a day, such as pears, apples or plums (you will have to eat more vegetables to compensate). After four weeks, eat no more than three pieces of organic fruit per day.

- **Nuts and seeds.** You can eat sunflower, pumpkin and sesame seeds. Ideally nuts should be freshly shelled – don't eat any shelled nuts that smell musty. Coconut, walnuts, almonds and cashews are good choices.

- **Legumes.** Include beans, lentils, chickpeas (including hummus) and soya products, such as tofu or soya cheese.

- **Dairy and eggs.** Restrict your intake of milk, which contains the milk sugar lactose, and try to stick to organic products. Live 'bio' yoghurt is the best way to eat dairy. Cottage cheese is fine and eggs may be eaten too.

- **Oils.** Use only unrefined, organic, cold-pressed olive, sunflower, safflower, soya, sesame, corn or canola oil.

- **Drinks.** Drink natural spring/mineral or filtered tap water. Herb teas such as chamomile, peppermint and ginger are good. Exclude fruit juices for three weeks or so and dilute vegetable juices 1:1 with water.

Here are the foods and drinks you'll need to avoid.

- **Sugar and refined carbohydrates**. These encourage unwelcome bacteria. Look out for the following. White and brown sugar and foods listed as containing added sucrose, fructose, glucose, dextrose, corn syrup or maltose. Honey, treacle, molasses, caramel or maple and other syrups. Cakes, biscuits, baked goods such as pastries should be avoided alongside puddings, ice cream, chocolate or other sweets. Alcoholic drinks. White flour, white rice and non-wholemeal pasta. Read labels and avoid processed foods containing sugars.

- **Yeast-containing foods**. You are likely to be sensitive to yeasts and any moulds that might be in your food. Leavened bread, rolls or pizza. Alcoholic drinks (again) or other fermented products, including vinegar, pickles, soy sauce or miso. Cheeses, buttermilk or sour cream. Hydrolysed vegetable protein or malted products. Yeast extracts, such as Marmite, Vegemite or Bovril, or other gravy mixes. Foods that may be contaminated with mould include musty-smelling nuts, mushrooms, grapes, dried fruits and fruit skins.

- **Additives**. Always check the ingredients on food labels. Avoid yeast, sugar, malt, vinegar, citric acid (for instance, in drinks or tinned tomatoes), monosodium glutamate (aka flavour enhancer E621, found in Chinese food and many processed or packaged foods). Also avoid peanuts and pistachio nuts.

- **Drinks**. Cut out all black tea, coffee and fizzy drinks, and flavoured 'squashes'.

- **Sweetners**. Cutting out sugar will enable you to re-educate your palate to enjoy more subtle flavours in food, while sweeteners simply keep you wanting an extreme level of sweetness. It is important that you learn good habits from this diet and do not fall back into the sugar habit.

PROBIOTICS – THE FRIENDLY FLORA

We have more bacteria in our bodies than there have ever been people on the planet. And most of these bacteria exist in the intestinal tract. But a diet of heavily processed foods can seriously limit the good 'probiotic' bacteria or friendly flora that keep the gut healthy and prevent the kind

---

of problems – wind, variable stools, fatigue and even skin conditions such as eczema – that occur when hostile bacteria are allowed to proliferate. Many, many patients find these symptoms are accompanied by what I call 'brain fog' – a feeling that their brain is all fogged up. Without a doubt, dysbiosis may affect cognitive ability.

Friendly flora inhibit the multiplication of unfriendly bacteria and yeasts in the gut. They also help to make vitamins, so they have a 'symbiotic' relationship with us. We provide them with an environment and food source, they protect us from unhealthy flora and produce valuable nutrients for us. Certain things are known to aggravate bad bacteria: antibiotics are a common culprit, generally killing off *all* bacteria, including the friendly strains, and the absence of these encourages the baddies to recolonise with a vengeance. Some women will recognise that they get vaginal thrush after taking antibiotics, and many people may have had disturbed intestinal function when taking antibiotics. (If you've been prescribed them, however, you do need to take them!) Another factor in the proliferation of yeasts is a diet rich in sugars or anything fermented (such as vinegar, wine, pickles and yeast spreads, if eaten very regularly) – so these are all things to consume only from time to time.

Very occasionally I will recommend the use of a systemic anti-fungal treatment such as Nystatin for fungal-type gut dysbiosis, but I prefer, whenever possible, to prescribe natural probiotic treatments alongside dietary advice. I recommend a supplement containing 4 million live lactobacillus bugs per capsule. I also encourage the use of fresh and ideally raw garlic, which is a wonderful anti-fungal remedy. Crush it into salad and eat it straight away. Crushing and mixing with olive oil also makes the garlic much more palatable. Raw whole cloves can give you nasty heartburn, so I don't recommend you eat them this way.

Grapefruit seed extract and the herb berberis (in supplement form) also help to rebalance the gut.

Again, don't self-medicate. Seek medical or naturopathic advice. And remember that anything you take must be justified and taken for a limited period only. I often see people who have been taking a great list of herbals/supplements, without a clear indication of why. Don't do it.

WHAT ABOUT CANDIDA?

So-called 'candida' provides another good example of how important it is to understand human health in its entirety. When Jo came to see me for the first time, she asked, as so many people do: 'I wonder if I've got candida?' (A senior diplomat, Jo had come to see me from her post abroad, on a flying visit to London.) Like many patients, she'd wondered about candida because she was experiencing wind, abdominal bloating and vaginal thrush. But it never pays to jump to conclusions about your health. All symptoms and changes in your health must be properly evaluated (in consultation with your own doctor). Symptoms associated with gut dysbiosis can have various physical causes – some of them serious – and investigation mustn't be delayed while seeking complementary approaches. Generally, the two types of treatment can go hand in hand.

Candida albicans is a yeast that occurs naturally in the human gut or female vagina, and sometimes in sweaty skin folds – where it is delightfully named 'runner's crutch'. Many women are all too familiar with the irritation and white discharge of vaginal thrush, so-called because the white colonies of the yeast appear on the vaginal walls like the speckles of a thrush's breast. Candida may also overgrow in the gut, producing the huge range of gut dysbiosis symptoms I have already mentioned.

If candida overgrows, there will be underlying causes that have to be found. For recurrent thrush, for example, diabetes must be excluded, as both thrush and skin-fold fungal infections are more common in diabetics. Anaemia is another trigger, along with iron deficiency and more serious culprits, which doctors will test for.

As I told Jo, there are a number of points to remember regarding gut dysbiosis and its role in human health:

• Although the mechanisms are not fully understood, healthy gut flora are beneficial to human health.

• Unhealthy gut flora may be fungal or bacterial.

• Fungal-type dysbiosis is a relatively common condition, with symptoms like lethargy, wind and bloating, feeling tired after meals, and in both sexes perineal irritation; and in women, it may be associated with vaginal thrush.

With most people, the condition reflects their dietary habits, and a change of diet is the solution.

As she left for a shopping spree and subsequent dash to the airport, Jo understood the issues involved far better. Treating her thrush was a straightforward, conventional medical matter, but correcting the gut dysbiosis is the only way to regain full health in both the gut flora and the rest of the body. Jo duly took my dietary guidelines with her and resolved to see a doctor if her symptoms did not settle entirely.

Gut dysbiosis and IBS: are they the same?

If you have been diagnosed with irritable bowel syndrome (IBS), you might now be thinking that fungal-type gut dysbiosis might be the problem. IBS, however – which is characterised by irregular bowel habit, alternating diarrhoea and constipation, pain, bloating and the like – is a *syndrome*, a collection of symptoms which can be caused by a great many factors. It is not a condition in itself, to be treated in isolation. It's a functional disorder, and people should not be labelled as IBS sufferers until physical causes have been ruled out.

IBS is, as we saw earlier, very common. One particular patient came to see me with classic symptoms. He had a longstanding history of IBS. As an accountant he was suffering 'year end' stress and put his changed bowel habit down to this. As I always do, I listened to his story and examined him, ascertaining whether blood or slime had been passed recently, if there had been any weight loss, or if there was a family history of bowel cancer or polyps. Suspicions aroused, I ordered immediate gastroenterological investigations, as I was concerned that his symptoms indicated something more serious than functional IBS. I was right, and my patient was admitted to hospital and prepared for surgery. Luckily, we were in time. Both doctors and patients must take bowel symptoms seriously. Remember that both functional and serious conditions can coexist. Never 'put up' with symptoms. If you are not well despite a healthy lifestyle, you must go back and tell your doctor. In any case, this patient's story reveals how IBS is, emphatically, a collection of symptoms, and physical pathology must not be ruled out.

Fungal-type gut dysbiosis is a distinct condition. It is quite common, as the trend towards eating refined carbohydrates, sugary snacks (even if they *are* marked as 'healthy') and fizzy sugary drinks has been a steady one. Recent courses of antibiotics, especially for long periods, may also disturb gut flora. Living alone, erratic lifestyle and work, and family pressures all conspire to disrupt healthy eating and lifestyle. Yet it's precisely that kind of eating and living that will clear up fungal-type dysbiosis.

To sum up regarding gut dysbiosis:

1. Do not assume from your reading or internet surfing that your fatigue, abdominal symptoms or whatever are down to an overgrowth of candida. It may well not be, and delays in diagnosis can be dangerous.

2. Be properly medically investigated and encourage communication between your doctor and naturopath.

Only having considered the relevant investigations and blood tests, and eliminated other potential causes of symptoms, can the treatment of gut dysbiosis begin. Following the low-sugar, low-yeast anti-dysbiosis diet (page 136) is the first, vital step. Cutting out fermented foods will lessen the symptoms, and reducing the intake of sugars helps starve out the unhealthy fungi and yeast organisms. I always stress to patients that this is a mixed, varied, non-vegetarian diet, and does not exclude any major food groups, although vegetarian versions will achieve the same results.

When you have followed the anti-dysbiosis diet for three to four weeks, it's sensible to review your progress and what you have achieved in terms of wellbeing. I would ask a person to see me after this period to discuss how to consolidate a healthier approach to eating. It's also very important to learn and understand why you feel better because this will help maintain the improvement. I would then gradually broaden the diet, moving towards the McManners Method Diet for long-term maintenance of good health.

With any diet, there are three stages:

1. Induction

This creates the initial changes that are necessary to start the process of improving health. With the anti-dysbiosis diet, I would expect an improvement in symptoms and wellbeing within three weeks or so.

2. Consolidation

It is then vital to continue any dietary regime to broaden the diet, to continue learning, to make plans for a longer-term change in diet, to enjoy and be interested in foods that maintain health and wellbeing. A healthy way of eating is not just a 'stick-on', temporary experiment. A person may feel better for three weeks or so, but if they go back to their old ways, symptoms of ill health will return.

3. Maintenance

Establishing changes and making the benefits permanent requires a long-haul dietary effort. But it's nothing like the imposition of the first and, to a lesser extent, the second stage. When enjoying a wide and varied healthy diet and improved health and wellbeing becomes a habit, you'll know it has become a permanent part of your life.

CHAPTER 12

Activity

Exercise is essential to physical health. Simply put, evolution insists on it. Our physiologies evolved to match a far more active lifestyle than the one we typically enjoy today. For millions of years, gathering the bare necessities of life involved hours of effort on a daily basis, punctuated by periods of particularly intense physical stress or activity. Even a hundred years ago, most people walked, carried, climbed and expended sheer elbow grease much more than today.

We're not built to sit around all day, and your body doesn't like it if that's all you do. The growing problem with obesity in the US, UK, Australia, and many other developed nations, is due to lower activity levels, not just, as many people believe, our diets. Although junk food has a lot to answer for, most of us are actually eating less than our ancestors. Low activity levels also lead to low bone density and a risk of osteoporosis, a high ratio of fat to muscle and an increased risk of getting a number of different degenerative diseases such as diabetes and arteriosclerosis. That's why your activity level is probably the most important influence on the physical corner of your triangle of health.

Of course, most people are well aware that being a couch potato is 'a bad thing', and exercise is 'a good thing'. But how do you know whether you're doing enough exercise, and, just as importantly, whether you're doing the right kind of exercise? Think about whether your activity level and the type of exercise you're doing are building or draining your reserves of physical health.

■ Lowdown on exercise

- Do you know the difference between aerobic and anaerobic exercise?

- Do you do aerobic exercise at least three times a week for at least 20 to 30 minutes per session?

- Do you know why it's important to take load-bearing exercise?

- Do you do any activities to improve your strength, flexibility, suppleness, posture or co-ordination?

■ What's the difference between aerobic and anaerobic exercise?

Aerobic exercise is any activity that raises your heart and breathing rate, generally making you sweat. Assuming that you do at least 20 to 30 minutes or so at a time, aerobic exercise conditions your cardiovascular and respiratory systems, burns calories and builds endurance and stamina – in short, it gets you fit.

Activities that fall into this category include jogging, swimming and walking (if done at a fast enough pace), rowing, cycling, cross-country skiing, skipping, dancing, climbing stairs and aerobics exercises. Surprisingly, sports like football, tennis or squash often have limited aerobic value because they tend to involve short, sharp bursts of activity, whereas aerobic exercise is all about continuous effort.

Activities that involve intense bursts of effort rather than sustained huffing and puffing are called anaerobic. These types of exercise tend to be good for toning and building muscles, increasing strength and speed, and/or for stretching and increasing flexibility and suppleness. Activities in this category include weight training, floor training (press-ups, sit-ups, squat thrusts and the like). Some activities, such as kick-boxing and circuit training, involve anaerobic activities done continuously and interspersed with aerobic bits, to produce a sort of aerobic/anaerobic hybrid.

■ How's your aerobic workout?

You need to exercise aerobically for at least 20 to 30 minutes to benefit your cardiovascular system, and you should be doing at least three such sessions per week to stay in shape and maintain fitness. This isn't as hard as it may sound. Walking fast enough and pushing yourself to keep your heart rate raised is an 'easy' exercise that counts (see page 152).

■ Are you doing any load-bearing exercise?

Load-bearing exercise – that is, exercise that involves putting weight or stress on your bones and joints, such as walking, running, low-impact aerobics, dancing or energetic yoga – can help reduce and even help reverse age-related muscle wastage and bone loss. If you're not doing any load-bearing activities you are increasing your risk of developing osteoporosis and muscle wastage in later life. It is this combination that reduces mobility in older age and increases the chances of falls and fractures. A fall is often the crisis event that robs a person of their independence – so keep active!

■ Are you exercising to improve your strength, flexibility, suppleness, posture or co-ordination?

Aerobic fitness is only one aspect of physical health. To properly maintain it, you need an integrated exercise programme that includes anaerobic exercises.

I count myself lucky to have been a very active person ever since I was a child. Lucky, because it means that I got into the habit of exercising a long time ago; and it's a habit that's now deeply ingrained, and a perfectly natural part of my life.

Here's an example of the exercise I take in a typical week. You may like to keep your own exercise diary for a few days to monitor your activity levels. Treat it like your food diary. Use it to see what you are doing (and what you're not!). The information in this chapter and in Chapter 13 will take you a step further. Why not try out some new forms of exercise? Even if you do exercise regularly, doing the same routine week in, week out, can be dull, and will be less benficial for your structural health than a range of activities.

I start every day with a good stretch – usually a few rounds of the yoga sun salutation (see page 165). In addition to this, I look after my animals, walk and swim. Although I do not attend many exercise 'classes', my activity level is, I consider, very adequate and I feel incredibly fit and strong.

Monday: Walked 3 miles briskly in the woods groomed two horses vigorously, and rode one of them for an hour.

Tuesday and Wednesday: These are the days I work in London. In theory I could do very little exercise while ensconced in my clinic. So I get off the Underground several stops too soon and walk briskly for one and a half miles. I do the same walk back in the evening, usually at high speed so as not to miss my train. Between patients, I make a point of walking fast up two flights of stairs so that I am not stuck in my seat all day long. This is something I have recommended to a number of time-poor patients, who say they simply cannot fit exercise into their busy working day. Five minutes of stair climbing every hour adds up to a neat 40 minutes over the course of an average working day!

Thursday: Walked about 3 miles doing outdoor chores and looking after my horses; played tennis with a friend.

Friday: Rode one of the horses for one and a half hours. I recommend riding to any woman wanting to keep in shape – a rising trot is a great waist and bottom trimmer! (Riding also gives me very good 'thinking time'!)

Saturday: Took my youngest son to a swimming lesson, so had a 40-minute swim while I was there. Sometimes I will use the gym equipment during his lesson.

Sunday: Walked with the family.

Getting the exercise habit really is the best way to build up your reserves of physical health. But all too few of my patients are lucky enough to have the exercise habit already – they have to develop it from scratch, which isn't an easy task. It takes willpower and effort, but the rewards are enormous. Hopefully you'll remember that my number one rule about diet and nutrition was 'Enjoy Your Food!' Well, my number one rule about exercise is: Enjoy Yourself!

Exercise isn't supposed to be a form of self-flagellation, where the more you suffer the worthier it makes you.

In fact, along with food, exercise shares the marvellous twin properties of being good for you and being immensely enjoyable. It's true that there will be some hard graft to start with if your activity levels are low, or you feel you've let yourself get badly out of shape. But in a surprisingly short time you could be experiencing for yourself the many and varied reasons so many people love to exercise.

MOVING STORY

Whole books could be written on the multiple physical, physiological and psychological benefits of exercise, but I'm just going to give you a brief rundown here.

- Exercise boosts your cardiovascular health. It strengthens your heart so that it can pump more blood with each stroke and therefore has to pump less. It may reduce the build-up of cholesterol deposits that cause arteriosclerosis, and lowers the level of LDL cholesterol – the harmful kind – in your bloodstream. It may also lower blood pressure and helps to regulate clotting factors in the blood. All in all, appropriate exercise significantly reduces the risk of heart attacks, strokes, aneurysms, blood clots and just about every other form of cardiovascular disease you can think of.

- It improves your respiratory health, helping you to breathe more deeply and efficiently, boosting circulation to all parts of the lungs and therefore the oxygen supply to the rest of the body – including your brain. People who walk at least a mile a day are more alert and work more efficiently. I feel great when I get to my clinic after a good walk.

- Exercise boosts your immune system, helping you to fight illness and reducing your risk of developing a range of infectious and degenerative diseases, from colds and flu to cancer, diabetes and osteoporosis.

- It helps you to lose weight and keep it off permanently. Regular exercise actually changes the balance of tissues in your body. It improves your 'body composition' – giving you a higher ratio of muscle to fat – and this increases your basal metabolic rate (the rate at which you burn calories), so the calories you eat are less likely to end up being laid down as fat, and you can eat more without putting on weight. Housewives in the 1950s, who had to manage without our labour-saving devices, ate more calories than women today but were slimmer.

- Exercise gives you strength, suppleness and endurance.

- It gives you more energy for physical tasks such as gardening or housework, as well as mental work. We all know we perform better at work when we have more energy – even if we do a desk job.

- Exercise makes you a better lover, with more sexual energy, a higher libido, greater endurance and lower risk of impotence or other sexual problems.

- It also makes you look better and younger, and feel more positive about yourself.

- It boosts confidence and assertiveness.

- It relieves stress and, because of the endorphins or 'feelgood' hormones it releases, it improves mood and can help beat depression.

Patients are often quick to tell me that they've just joined the gym, and that this year they'll make good on their New Year's resolution to get fit. But it's now well known that gyms make most of their money selling expensive annual memberships to people who stop going after a few weeks. Like dieting, taking up exercise is doomed to failure when it's treated as an 'add-on', a quick fix, a fad. As with your diet and nutrition, you need to make healthy principles a permanent and enjoyable part of your life. In the case of exercise, this means becoming a more active person, walking more, running more, climbing more stairs. Obviously I'm not suggesting that you should change your whole outlook and lifestyle overnight, but I am saying that you may well need to make long-term, permanent changes, which is where the 'habit' comes in.

Make exercise a habit by including walking, stair-climbing, running and cycling as part of your journey to work – rather than using a car or public transport. It takes a bit of organisation, but you can walk, cycle or run to work at least some of the time or for part of the journey, say to and from the railway station, with your work clothes in a small backpack. You can have a quick wash and change when you get there – or keep your suit on a hanger at work. Exercise as transportation means you have to do it. You could also join a gym close to work, and to avoid the lunchtime exercise rush, come to work earlier and go before work. This is preferable to going at the end of the day when your body (not to mention your mind) may invent all sorts of reasons to be too tired to work out – and will interfere with after-work social life. By making an exercise an enjoyable routine, you develop a really good habit.

Naturopathy and exercise

Exercise is an essentially naturopathic activity, because it involves all aspects of a person's health. In some ways it's one of the best holistic treatments available, as a healthy diet is necessary if you're to refuel your energy, and rest is required to recharge your psychological batteries. But an important and often overlooked aspect of naturopathy is its emphasis on the simple delights of fresh air, sunlight and being outside in general (things we'll be talking about in the next chapter) – so I always encourage patients to get outside whenever they can. Jogging, cycling, walking, riding and rowing are all good opportunities to get out in the open air and make your exercise truly naturopathic. But it is also crucial that you choose activities you will enjoy, as you are far more likely to stick to something *you* find fun.

As well as enjoying what you do, and doing it outside whenever you can, I recommend going for variety in your workout. Just as your diet should be varied to supply a full array of nutrients, your exercise programme should be varied to cover the four aspects of fitness:

- Flexibility

- Strength

- Aerobic fitness

- Endurance

A combination of aerobic exercises for fitness and health, and anaerobic exercises for toning, suppleness and relaxation, will allow you to achieve this.

When planning your new programme, think back about what you have enjoyed doing in the past. When I ask patients about their exercise history, I am not just looking for clues about their current level of fitness. I also want to know what makes them tick.

For instance, if someone preferred solitary sports while they were at school, like cross-country running, they're more likely to go for exercise they can do on their own, like cycling or jogging. If they were more of a team sports person, enjoying football or netball, for instance, they might prefer a different mix of activities like squash or cricket.

What sort of (non-sporting) pastimes do you enjoy? Maybe there's a way to combine them with some exercise. Were you keen on a particular sport when you were at school? Maybe you could get involved in it again. How do your preferences match up with your local amenities? Maybe you live near a park, close to stables or opposite a gym. You're a lot more likely to make a habit of an activity you can do locally.

Aerobic activities

Many people find even the thought of aerobic exercise exhausting, and of course it *is* tiring – that is the point of it. But aerobic exercise is one of those things that gets easier the more you do it, and I'm not just talking about your time over a certain course or how long you can run/row/ski/skip for. Finding the energy and motivation to go and do some exercise becomes easier. You should finish feeling energised and happier. Cooling down afterwards becomes easier. Even finding the time for exercise in your busy schedule becomes easier – because your body starts to yearn for it. The converse, of course, is that the less exercise you do the harder it gets, and the less regular you are about doing it, the harder it gets – another good reason for making exercise a habit.

Types of aerobic exercise You're really spoiled for choice here – there are many great forms of aerobic exercise, starting with plain and simple (as well as enjoyable and effective) walking.

- **Walking** is the most accessible form of aerobic activity, and also one of the safest. Beyond a pair of sturdy shoes, preferably with good ankle support, you don't need any special equipment and you can do it anywhere – although obviously scenic locations are more interesting than the local high street. The main drawback of walking as exercise is that it's generally low intensity. For it to be more valuable as an aerobic exercise, you need to do a relatively long, uninterrupted walk at a sustained pace. Work up to covering about 3 miles in 45 minutes to start with. Once you can manage this you can move on to walking further, faster or over more challenging terrain – not just on the flat but coping with inclines as well. Just about anybody can make walking a valid exercise. One woman I know who is approaching 100 years old walks around her ground floor for five minutes or so every hour. This is tremendous as it combats statis and the risk of thrombosis in her legs, improves her circulation and focuses her mind – and she is still a quickwitted card player!

  Never wear ankle weights. Walking and running are natural exercises, and should not be complicated with unnatural devices like ankle weights, weights held in the hands or weights in backpacks – which do no good. Soldiers training for combat load themselves up for battle runs because this is what they have to be able to do. Weight training is a separate type of exercise and should be done exclusively in special weight-training sessions.

- **Running/jogging** are almost as accessible as walking. Running has the advantage of being a more intense form of exercise, but does stress the body (it's what's called a 'high-impact' activity). Running for more than 20 minutes gives a good aerobic workout, burning calories and increasing your fitness levels faster than most other activities, but you must take precautions to minimise the possibility of damaging your body. Wear high-quality specialist running shoes and replace them as soon as they start to wear out. Women should wear sports bras. Run on soft surfaces such as grass, sand, dirt or a track if at all possible. If it isn't, remember that tarmac is better than concrete, which creates a pounding effect on the feet, ankles and lower back, and can lead to strain injuries – especially if you are overweight or not wearing the correct shoes (or even new shoes you're not yet used to).

If you want to avoid the vagaries of the weather, or don't have anywhere suitable for jogging nearby (it's best to avoid running alongside traffic, as you'll breathe in too many fumes), you could try running on a treadmill in the gym. Bear in mind, however, that this is easier than the real thing, so you should build up to setting the treadmill at a slight incline.

- **Swimming** is a lower-intensity activity than running, but it's a lot easier on the joints and gives you an all-over workout. It's great for everyone but is particularly suitable for older people or anyone with structural problems such as back pain or arthritis. Use well-fitting goggles to avoid eye problems from chlorinated water (which can cause a lot of irritation). The crawl (freestyle) is the most aerobic stroke, but it can take some skill to master the breathing required. Try to turn your head both ways to avoid getting neck ache. Some swimming lessons would be a good idea to make sure you don't develop long-term bad habits. Many ladies swim breaststroke holding their head out of the water and this can be a strain on the neck – even though it doesn't spoil the make-up! So try not to hold the head up at a sharp angle to the upper back.

- **Cycling** obviously requires some special equipment, in the form of a bike and helmet. And, like walking, it needs to be done at a relatively high level of intensity to give a good aerobic workout (over 10 mph). It is much easier on the knees than jogging, however, strengthens the legs at the same time, and can be a good exercise for those recovering from knee or leg problems. Cycling is a brilliant way to get out and about if you have access to the countryside, but for those worried about dangerous roads, a stationary bike may be a better and safer option.

- **Dancing** is a personal favourite of mine, as I spent much of my childhood training to be a dancer. But it's also an underrated form of aerobic exercise with loads of fringe benefits. Not only does it provide a great aerobic workout, it also improves postural awareness, fine control of muscles and joints, co-ordination, balance, flexibility and breathing. But better than any of these, it's fun! The music and the feeling of energy and liberation make dancing a great tonic for the soul as well as the body. In practical terms, dancing is extremely accessible – anyone can do it at any time. It just needs music and floor space. Many people like to dance with other people, though – hence the popularity of salsa, aerobics classes, 'dancercise', line dancing and so on. The only problem is that dancing is traditionally thought of as being a bit 'sissy', which tends to put men off. Hopefully the growing popularity of salsa and similar forms of dance is counteracting this perception. Many of my patients – young and not so young – have met this way.

- **Cross-country skiing, rowing and other exercises** are good all-round aerobic exercises, but most people won't have access to the real things. Cross-country skiing machines are said to provide the best all-round workouts, but, like rowing machines, they require a bit of expertise to use properly. Rowing machines in particular can cause back problems if not used properly. Other good exercises include stair-machines (high-intensity stuff – not for the faint of heart) and skipping, which requires little equipment and boosts co-ordination as well as giving a good arm and leg workout, but is tough to keep up for long enough. Book a few sessions with a personal trainer – most gyms have them – so you know you are using the equipment correctly (adopting the wrong technique or posture can do you more harm than good). Ask the gym about their trainers' qualifications, as there may be large variations in levels of competence. Some are qualified to a level that enables them to accept medical referrals for some conditions, which is reassuring.

Take due care   Aerobic exercise puts stress on your heart and circulation, and, depending on the activity, various joints, tendons, bones and muscles. You must be careful and apply some common sense when doing it.

- **Check with your doctor before exercising**, especially if you've got a history of cardiovascular problems, or if there's a family history of problems, or if you're overweight or recovering from injury or illness.

- **Stop immediately if you feel light-headed** or develop pain in your chest or arm or headaches. Go and see a doctor immediately.

- **Listen to your body** – if your muscles or joints start to ache continuously (beyond the stiffness you can expect when you begin exercising) or you suffer joint swelling, then switch to a different form of exercise and take the strain off them. Again, seek medical advice.

- **Don't exercise when unwell.** Although being fit will help stop you becoming unwell, and increase the speed at which you get better, you must not exercise while you're actually below par or feel that you may be developing a cold or flu, for example. If you exercise when you have a viral infection, it can actually lead to serious complications. When you are unwell, rest: you need to draw on your reserves of health to get better again.

Too many people – particularly men – leap feet first into an exercise programme rather than building up slowly. They may have done lots of exercise in the past and expect to start again where they left off, or they may simply be busy people who want results fast.

Unfortunately, exercise doesn't work like this, and jumping the gun or literally running before you can walk can have negative consequences. Failure to reach overambitious targets could put you off exercise before you've really begun. Even worse, loading your body with too much stress all at once could lead to an injury.

Start slow   Don't be too ambitious to start with. Set realistic goals, and build up gradually but steadily – the frequency of exercise is initially more important than the intensity.

- If you have previously had very low activity levels or are overweight, consider low-impact, low-intensity exercises first – walking, swimming and cycling are all good options.

- If you want to jog, build up to a full session by interspersing five-minute bursts of jogging with two minutes of walking. Aim to do 10 minutes the first time, 15 minutes the second time and so on.

- Similarly, for swimming, intersperse crawl with breaststroke; for cycling, particularly on a stationary bike where the readout shows your speed or rate of work, intersperse gentle with more intense cycling.

- Plan regular sessions, but don't be derailed by your own schedule. As with dieting, the occasional lapse shouldn't put you off altogether. If you miss a planned session, don't worry about it – simply go the next day.

The start slow rule applies to individual exercise sessions as well – you should always warm up before launching into aerobic or any other type of exercise. Stretching is a worthwhile activity in itself, although it may be of comparatively little use in preventing injury. To warm up properly you need to do a slow version of the exercise you're about to undertake, for at least five minutes.

Never say never Research shows that you can enjoy the health benefits of exercise whatever your age, and that it's never too late to start. Load-bearing exercise in particular can help reduce and even reverse to some extent age-related muscle wastage and bone loss. Obviously, the older you are or the more complicated your medical history, the more careful you need to be about getting initial medical assessment and advice, monitoring your progress, listening to your body and getting appropriate supervision.

Fight boredom A common complaint about exercise – especially aerobic exercise or gym workouts – is that it's boring. This is a real problem, and is one of the biggest reasons people either give up or never take up regular exercise. There are all sorts of ways you can liven up an exercise session and make working out more enjoyable.

- **Follow naturopathic principles**, which emphasise the simple sensory pleasures of the world around us. If you're open to your surroundings, for instance, a brisk aerobic walk through busy city streets or a green country lane can become a moveable feast of colour, light, sound and smells.

- **Add music.** Aerobics classes use dance soundtracks to provide a rhythm for the movement, and to energise, entertain and help participants keep up the pace. A personal soundtrack can liven up your workout in the same way.

- **Multi-task.** If you're working out on a stationary bike or other machine, try positioning it in front of a television or a book or newspaper stand, or turn on the radio.

ACTIVITY

- Make your days active – even if it's only walking partway to work or running up and down stairs

- Find a form of aerobic exercise that's enjoyable for you

- Check with your GP before starting anything new if you are unfit, overweight or have a health concern

- Combine aerobic exercise with anaerobic exercise for strength and flexibility (see Chapter 13)

Body structure

How you hold and use your body – your posture, strength and flexibility – have a huge impact on your health, affecting everything from back pain to headaches and IBS. Think about the following questions. Maybe they don't seem important – but read further and you'll see just how important they are.

In this chapter, as well as encouraging you to think about your posture and your physical environment, I'll be discussing some simple stretches and exercises to get your body back on track, and some longer-term activities that are particularly good for posture and structural strength. If you have a sedentary job in an office or perform any kind of repetitive movement, these exercises are particularly important, but it's important for everyone to be aware of these aspects of their health and possible causes of problems. You can be sedentary at home, too!

■ Posture and ergonomics

- Do you pay much attention to your posture?

- Does your posture have the following characteristics? Viewed from the side, it looks as though there is a straight line through your head, spine and legs; an open-shouldered stance. And when seated, your head is directly over your chest and pelvis and your arms and legs are bent at right angles

- Does your posture have any of these characteristics? Head held in front of the rest of body, causing neck to protrude forwards; rest of the upper body also thrust forward and buttocks thrust backwards

- Do you have a rounded back and hunched shoulders?

- Do you have a pot belly?

- Do you work in an office or other job where you spend much of the time sitting down?

- How often do you get up and walk around or stretch?

- Does your job involve repetitive movements, such as typing?

- What's your work environment like?

■ Are you aware of your posture?

Many people are not very aware of their posture, and if it's not good, they often wait until it's too late and they're suffering back pain, headaches and other problems as a result. Take a moment to evaluate your own posture. Stand in front of a mirror and look at the way you hold your body. Move a chair in front of the mirror and, using a hand mirror to see your reflection, see what you look like sitting down, especially if this is what you do all day at work.

HOW YOU HOLD YOURSELF

Posture is a crucial aspect of physical health because of its strong influence on the structural elements of your body. The way you hold yourself physically changes the alignments and relationships of the bones, joints, muscles, ligaments and tendons. It changes the dimensions of your chest and determines how effectively you breathe. It also directly affects the blood vessels and therefore blood flow; the nerves and therefore nervous functions such as pain, sensation and muscular control; the digestive tract and therefore digestion and bowel habit. In fact it affects, directly or indirectly, almost every organ, tissue and system of the body.

Poor posture has a constant and serious debilitating influence on the rest of your system. It can sap your reserves of health and weaken your defences against disease; place direct strain on the structural elements of your body, interfering with breathing, digestion, blood flow and other processes; and affect you psychologically and spiritually. A tired, depressed, subdued posture may be closely tied to low energy levels and a depressed, negative or defensive outlook on life.

■ Do you have all the signs of good posture?

Good posture is often described as looking as if a string is attached to the top of the head, pulling the rest of the body into line below it. Although your spine follows natural curves, if looked at side on, it should be possible to imagine a straight line through your head, spine, pelvis and legs (see the illustration opposite).

An open-shouldered rather than round-shouldered stance encourages diaphragmatic breathing, where the diaphragm is the main muscle driving inspiration. You can check this by watching yourself in the mirror while breathing naturally – it should be your belly rather than your chest that obviously expands with each breath. When lying down, you should see your abdomen gently rise and fall.

If your posture, standing and seated, does not match up to this description, you could be setting yourself up for – or already experiencing – the effects of poor posture.

■ Do you have any of the signs of poor posture?

The most characteristic sign of poor posture is to hold the head in front of the rest of the body. Sometimes the rest of the upper body is also thrust forward and the buttocks are thrust backwards to compensate, giving an almost duck-like profile (see the illustration opposite).

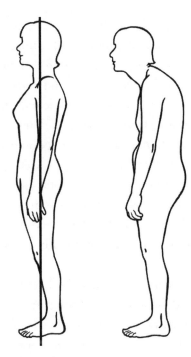

Correct (left) and incorrect posture (right)

This posture causes problems because the head is very heavy, and when it's not properly positioned with the whole body aligned underneath for support, it can place a lot of strain on the neck. The cervical vertebrae become misaligned, affecting the spinal nerves and blood vessels, sometimes leading to pins and needles, restricted neck mobility, stiffness, tension headaches and irritability. The forward neck posture is often associated with round shoulders and upper back, known as kyphosis (see below).

Poor posture is very common indeed, and unless instructed in good posture from an early age – for example, in dance or drama classes – many people will need assessment and postural advice. We walk around on two legs rather than the four 'legs' we were originally provided with, and this isn't the easiest of postures to cope with, so it is very easy to fall into bad habits without realising it. In the 1950s, my mother attended classes run by the Women's League of Health and Beauty which focused on good posture, training habits, exercise developing poise and elegant movement. Unfortunately, the 'liberation' of the 1960s stifled efforts of this sort and 'anything went'. But I can still remember the voice of my ballet teacher: 'Tummies in – bottoms in!' This posture encourages poise and graceful movement combined with developing the considerable strength that is required for controlled movement. To have posture, strength and control is a good feeling, and one I take immense pleasure in. Although I gave up dancing years ago, people still comment on my posture and movement, which came from my dance training.

You don't need to train in dance to have good posture, though. How we sit, stand and breathe all affect our health. It is well worth focusing on how we use and misuse our bodies. One of my patients is a venerable, extremely distinguished academic who has spent his working life labouring over large tomes in university libraries, and has developed hunched shoulders and a forward posture neck, which have prevented him from breathing properly and achieving full chest inflation.

He suffers from bronchial and other chest complaints, and each winter dreads inevitable and debilitating chest infections, which lay him low for several weeks at a time. Although he smoked as a young man, while fighting as an infantry officer throughout the Second World War, he hasn't touched a cigarette for over 50 years. It's his poor posture that has made him more vulnerable to chest infections, as it limits his chest expansion and he cannot clear mucus easily. The condition of his chest had deteriorated since he had to give up playing tennis, which had really helped to open up his shoulders and expand his ribcage. But my patient is a brilliant man, and years ago developed his own system of stretching exercises that he does every day, with the advice of a physio and exercise therapist. Modifying his exercise regime to encourage good posture has certainly helped him even further. He intends to live a very long time, and not succumb to a chest infection.

The Austrian naturopath Dr Franz Mayr observed and recorded types of poor posture and unhealthy habits of living. Our posture affects the tension of our muscles. Many will be familiar with neck tension and stiffness after hours of sitting (in the wrong posture) in their office. Most people's working lives are now spent sitting, often peering into a screen, typing and using the phone simultaneously. A long way indeed from the hunter-gatherer lifestyle! But there's no need to revert back to our distant ancestral past, although we do need to be aware of how we are misusing our bodies.

■ Do you have a rounded back and hunched shoulders?

These are signs of early kyphosis, or curvature of the thoracic spine, which impedes breathing and respiratory capacity. This is a surprisingly common postural mistake, often found in people who work at computers or are otherwise deskbound. It needs to be actively corrected – consider learning the Alexander Technique or take classes in yoga or Pilates (see pages 164–8 for more on all of these), all of which improve your consciousness of correct spinal alignment. Osteopathic assessment and an appropriate prescribed exercise regime will also help.

■ Do you have a pot belly?

A pot belly and poor abdominal muscle tone can cause you to stand with a pelvic tilt that thrusts the abdomen forwards while the rest of the upper body is displaced back to compensate. This can cause lower back pain, and impede diaphragmatic breathing. Pot bellies are normally caused by poor posture (especially among people who spend much of their time seated) and lack of exercise. People in some occupations, such as taxi or truck driving, have to take especial care.

Activities for flexibility, posture and balance

The following forms of exercise will increase your flexibility and improve your co-ordination and balance.

- **Stretching** is the simplest of this group of activities. Unlike many of the others, it generally requires little or no instruction, especially if you have been to exercise classes in the past. Nevertheless if you've got structural problems such as back pain or arthritis it's a good idea to be medically assessed first. Your doctor may suggest seeing a physiothera-pist, for example. I recommend doing stretching exercises from time to time throughout the day (see page 176); they're also a particularly good 'pick-me-up' in the morning and when you get home from work. Try doing stretches that counteract strain or tension caused by your normal posture.

QUICK WHOLE-BODY STRETCH

1. With your feet a 'hips' distance' apart, reach upwards as far as you can with both hands, and go up onto the tips of your toes and down again.

2. Rotate both arms forwards and backwards, brushing ears with upper arms. Don't forget to breathe!

3. Rotate upper body from the waist as far to either side as you can, keeping feet firmly on the floor. Do three to each side. Keep your bottom still while you do this.

4. Stretch calves by leaning forwards pushing against a wall to stretch the back of each leg at a time.

5. Stretch thighs: stand one-legged (holding on to a wall bar or a chair back for support), bend the other knee, hold your ankle and gently pull your foot towards your buttocks.

6. Stretch your hamstrings by sitting with legs stretched out, then slowly moving forwards to touch your toes with your fingertips. Your legs may be bent slightly. Only do what you can do comfortably. This will slowly improve.

7. Do a coiling and uncoiling exercise. Stand straight and roll head forward, rounding shoulders and gently curving spine down to touch fingers towards feet. Keep knees slightly bent. Then uncoil slowly back up again.

- **Yoga** is a very all-round, naturopathic activity. Its various forms make it suitable for all ages and body types, and I'm a big fan of it. As well as conditioning your muscles and joints and stretching your tendons and ligaments, it also focuses on breathing, meditation, calmness and relaxation. Although you need to go to classes to learn about it, it's important to practise at home on a regular basis. A lot depends on your teacher, and you may need to try several different teachers, or even different types of yoga, before you find one

A YOGA TASTER

The Sun Salutation

Follow the instructions below. Your movements should be slow and relaxed, and your breathing steady and in time with your movements.

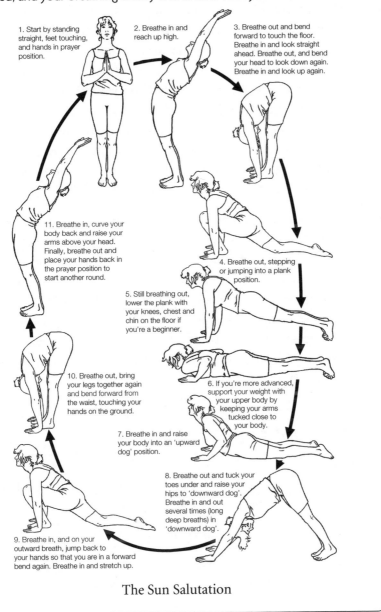

1. Start by standing straight, feet touching, and hands in prayer position.

2. Breathe in and reach up high.

3. Breathe out and bend forward to touch the floor. Breathe in and look straight ahead. Breathe out, and bend your head to look down again. Breathe in and look up again.

11. Breathe in, curve your body back and raise your arms above your head. Finally, breathe out and place your hands back in the prayer position to start another round.

4. Breathe out, stepping or jumping into a plank position.

5. Still breathing out, lower the plank with your knees, chest and chin on the floor if you're a beginner.

10. Breathe out, bring your legs together again and bend forward from the waist, touching your hands on the ground.

6. If you're more advanced, support your weight with your upper body by keeping your arms tucked close to your body.

7. Breathe in and raise your body into an 'upward dog' position.

8. Breathe out and tuck your toes under and raise your hips to 'downward dog'. Breathe in and out several times (long deep breaths) in 'downward dog'.

9. Breathe in, and on your outward breath, jump back to your hands so that you are in a forward bend again. Breathe in and stretch up.

The Sun Salutation

you're comfortable with and enjoy. As a general rule, hatha yoga is the most suitable for beginners. Avoid teachers who try to push you into difficult positions. Some one-to-one classes would be great if you can get them. The idea of yoga is that you do your own personal best. It is not a competitive sport!

- **Martial arts** include more good all-round activities, including judo, karate, kick-boxing, kung-fu, aikido, capoeira (Brazilian dance-fighting), tae kwon do and t'ai chi. Martial arts build self-confidence as well as flexibility and strength, but they can place more emphasis on the martial than the art. Again, a lot depends on your teacher/class, and you should shop around until you find the right one for you. I would recommend t'ai chi and capoeira as the most relaxing and least intimidating. I often recommend t'ai chi – often described as 'meditation in motion' – to slightly older people, although even the very young can get a great deal from it.

- **Pilates is a winner**. After all, an exercise routine has got to be pretty good when Hollywood stars swear by it. And since they, more than almost anyone, have to look wonderful while dealing with hugely demanding schedules, who better to follow? Pilates doesn't even feel like hard work, but it strengthens your core muscles – the ones that are hardest to reach using conventional forms of exercise – and it is particularly good for improving your breathing and posture and strengthening your back. It is also suitable for people of any age and, under appropriate instruction, even the very elderly can learn and benefit from Pilates exercise.

A PILATES TASTER

The Tree

This Pilates version of a classic yoga exercise will improve your posture by helping you learn to balance from within. In front of a mirror:

- Breathe in and lift and lengthen your spine.

- Breathe out, then pull your navel into your spine, putting your weight on to one leg and keeping your pelvis completely level.

- Lift the other leg off the floor, continuing to lengthen your waist on both sides (and keeping your pelvis level).

- Find your balance and breathe normally for a few breaths before returning the foot to the floor.

- Repeat five times per leg.

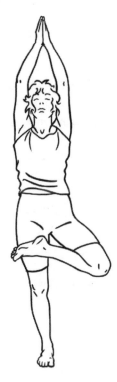

The Tree

The Classic Pilates Tummy Exercise

- Lie on your back with your pelvis neutral, so it's flat, not tilted.

- Breathe in fully.

- Breathe out, pull your navel into your spine and fold one knee at a time up on to your chest.

- Breathe in and with both hands take hold of your right leg under the thigh. Keep your elbows open and your breastbone soft. Your shoulder blades stay down into your back, and your neck is relaxed.

- Breathe out, pull your navel back to your spine and slowly straighten the left leg straight up into the air. Keep your back anchored into the floor. Do not arch it.

- Breathe in and bend the left knee back in to your chest. Change hands and hold your left thigh.

- Work up to repeating 10 times with each leg, keeping your back firmly anchored to the floor to protect your spine each time – this will tighten the very deepest of your abdominal muscles.

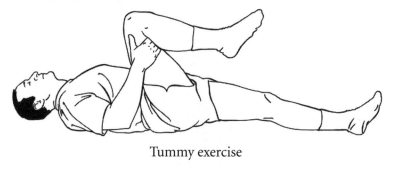

Tummy exercise

- **The Alexander Technique** is a venerable naturopathic therapy that teaches you to ease away from poor postural habits you may have begun in childhood by cultivating self-awareness. The brainchild of actor F. Matthias Alexander, it's extremely gentle and accessible to all ages and body types, and can have far-reaching positive health benefits. Essentially, it involves becoming aware of tensions in the body and, via specialised instruction, discovering the right way to move or stand. As with other forms of postural correction, this can have a dramatic impact on your wellbeing, as tension disappears and you begin to move around with ease. The effects can really be quite remarkable in terms of your wellbeing, as I found after my very first Alexander lesson.

Strength-building activities

Many women are put off forms of exercise that increase strength and muscle tone because they're worried they'll 'bulk up' and develop unfeminine contours. But working on your strength and muscle tone doesn't necessarily mean body-building. You won't develop bulging muscles unless you're trying really hard to do so. Body-building is big business and body builders eat a special high-protein diet and pump iron fairly intensively, using progressively heavier weights to bulk up. Your gym instructor or trainer will advise you on what is right for you and how you can increase the strength as well as the balance of all your muscle groups – for example, your back and your abdominal muscles. All too often people will focus on hundreds of 'abs' exercises, and will fail to include back exercises to balance the musculature of the whole trunk. You must exercise your body evenly.

- **Weight training** involves working muscles against resistance, helping to tone and strengthen them. It demands expert supervision at the beginning as it's very easy to strain something, whether you're a beginner or expert, unless you're carrying out weight-training exercises properly. You also won't get the full benefit of your effort if your technique is wrong. Beginners are best off starting with Nautilus or similar machines in a club. Don't buy a set of weights for home until you're serious about this form of exercise and you know what you're doing.

- **Floor work/callisthenics** works your muscles against the resistance of gravity, or each other, and is the classic type of workout that most of us used to do at school – press-ups, sit-ups, pull-ups, squat thrusts and star jumps. Why not stick with what you know? Apart from being excellent forms of exercise, callisthenics also require no equipment and can be done practically anywhere. You might find the prospect of sit-ups or press-ups daunting, but there are intermediate grades of intensity you can try. For instance, you can do press-ups from a kneeling position, which is a very good way of starting out, or standing up against a wall. Remember that it's more important to do each type of exercise slowly and properly than lots of times.

Cross-training

Remember: the key to good physical health is a rounded, varied exercise programme. Apart from maintaining your interest, there's also a good physiological reason for adopting a varied exercise programme. To increase levels of fitness and strength you need to challenge your body, working to performance levels just beyond its normal maximum. Your body, however, is cunningly designed to cope with changing demands and environments by adapting quickly, and altering its physiology to try to maintain stability. One example of this adaptability is the way your body responds to dieting. If you start to eat less, your body responds by downshifting its metabolism, so that it conserves energy and burns calories (and therefore fat) more slowly. This is why it can be hard to lose weight simply by eating less – you need to eat properly, but increase your activity levels as well so that your body cannot switch to energy conservation mode.

A similar process happens with exercise. If your body gets used to a certain physical load – a 30-minute run over the same course every two days, for instance – it will adapt so that it doesn't have to make significant physiological changes. Your workout will stop leading to improvements in fitness, strength and so on. To avoid this you need to vary both the type and intensity of exercise you do, through cross-training and rotation. Cross-training involves mixing different types of exercise – such as jogging one day, weight training the next, playing squash the day after. Activities that combine different forms of exercise come into their own here. Boxercise, martial arts and circuit training (doing a circuit of different floor work and weight-training activities in one session) are good examples. Rotation means varying the intensity of your exercise – for example, some days you do low-intensity exercise such as swimming, and others you'll do higher-intensity exercise, such as circuit training.

The one-hour window

Exercising speeds up your metabolism, as your body tries to meet the increased energy demands being made on it. Its metabolic 'thermostat' takes around an hour to reset to normal levels (less time the fitter you get), and this is a good time to eat because the nutrients from the food will be distributed and used in a healthier fashion than normal. Carbohydrates are less likely to be converted into fats, while protein is more likely to be diverted to your muscles than converted to fat. The hour after your workout is therefore a good 'window' for eating a healthy meal – ideally one with complex carbo-hydrates, and protein sources containing beneficial fats such as the essential fatty acids, and no saturated fats. A good example would be a bean salad with oily fish such as mackerel or wild salmon, rice and vegetables.

'BUT I HAVEN'T GOT TIME TO EXERCISE!'

A lot of my patients are very busy people, and the chances are that you too have a lot of demands on your time. You might agree in principle that doing more exercise would be a 'good thing', but who has the luxury of free time for the gym, pool and so on? Perhaps you're one of the many people who would say, 'I haven't got time to exercise!'

It's true that we only have a finite amount of time, and demands on it seem to be constantly increasing. By the time you get to the end of this book I'll have advised you to take more time out to shop, cook, eat, reflect, relax, stretch, get out into the countryside, walk in the garden, sleep, meditate, spend quality time as well as what I call 'ordinary time' with your family and friends, maybe get involved with your community, pursue your creative interests, get organised and interact with animals, all on top of your normal routine of work, childcare, housework and the rest! So how can you fit regular exercise in on top of this?

There's no simple answer to this problem. Better time management and learning not to take on too much can help reduce your workload (issues we'll be looking at in Chapter 19), but at heart it's a matter of priorities. Given the benefits of doing regular exercise and the risks associated with not doing it, exercise must rate as a high priority. It also may not be as disruptive to your lifestyle as you initially fear. Once it becomes a habit you're more likely to wonder how you managed without it. My advice? Just take the plunge – it's the only way to make it happen.

■ Do you work in an office where you are sitting down a lot?

This concern, and the ones that follow, are all to do with ergonomics – the study of how humans relate to their work environment, particularly in the physical sense. Most of us spend a lot of our lives at work, and the physical strains and constraints of these environments are some of the leading causes of poor posture, back pain, repetitive strain injuries and other problems that affect the physical corner of the triangle of total health.

How, and how much, we sit is a big issue for ergonomists. Most people's jobs these days involve a lot of sitting, and that poses a variety of problems. Inactivity is one of the most serious consequences of office work. Average activity levels are a fraction of what they were in times gone by, and as we've seen, a huge increase in gym membership doesn't always mean people are actually disciplined enough to use the gyms once they've paid up. Obesity, diabetes, cardiovascular disease and some cancers (including breast cancer) are all linked to low levels of activity, while weak muscles and inflexible joints, tendons and ligaments directly contribute to musculo-skeletal problems and risk of injury.

And that's not all. When we really do need to sit, our furniture often lets us down. Poorly designed seats and workstations give inadequate back support and force the body into bad postural habits for extended periods. Strain is placed on the neck and back, leading to back and joint pain, headaches and very often to the 'neck-forward' posture that so often leads to health problems (see the illustration on page 161).

Your eyes can also suffer if they are at the wrong level/distance in relation to your computer screen. This makes it hard for them to focus properly, and the eye muscles that change the shape of the lens will be constantly straining. Poor lighting makes the problem worse, while long periods of concentrated work without blinking can dry out the eyes, causing a different set of problems – irritation, redness and increased vulnerability to infection. Some people will need spectacles for computer work; if you have to squint and peer into your screen, you're bound to end up with poor posture. In the UK employers are required to monitor their employees' working conditions, but if you are self-employed or a home computer user, take care to have your eyes checked.

■ How often do you get up and walk around or stretch?

Prolonged sitting without moving the legs also increases the risk of circulatory problems such as deep-vein thrombosis (the so-called 'economy class syndrome', referring to the risk of it occurring on cramped planes), while lack of space and time for stretching or relaxation can exacerbate the problems described above. Make a point of getting up and walking around for at least five minutes every half-hour or so.

CHAINED TO A DESK

One of the most common consequences of poor posture is disturbed bowel habit. Jamie, a 29-year-old working in the newspaper industry, is a typical example. He came to see me because of chronic constipation that had been getting worse ever since he'd left university. He was surprised as he considered this to be a problem that affected only older people, and also because he was making a real effort to follow a healthy diet, which is pretty difficult amid the cut and thrust of a busy newsroom. He ate a good, varied selection of foods, including seeds, vegetable juice and plenty of fibre.

Discussing his past, I learned that at school and college he'd been very sporty, and captained the cricket and rugby teams. All this ground to a halt, however, when he became a journalist, and he now spent his days sitting in the newsroom peering into his screen. He had no time for the team sports that he used to be so keen on, and even at his young age the damage that was being done to his posture was apparent. He stooped, with his head slightly in front rather than in line with his body, and had the beginnings of round shoulders and a sway back.

Good physical posture and movement improve gut motility and promote regular bowel habit, but bad posture and inactivity have the opposite effect. Somehow we needed to get Jamie back into the active mode of his younger days, but working within the constraints of his office environment. First, I advised him to check the ergonomics of his working environment and discuss making changes to his seating arrangements with his boss. Secondly, I told him to spend five minutes out of every hour walking around his office focusing on his posture (as well as his work!). Over a 10-hour working day, that's nearly an hour of gentle exercise improving his posture and circulation. Lastly, I sent him to an osteopathic colleague to talk him through exercises to do at home and in the office. Over the next six weeks or so, his bowel habit improved significantly until he was no longer constipated.

Jamie's case emphasises the importance of the triangle of health. He already enjoyed a good diet (the biochemical corner), but needed help with the physical corner to get back on track.

■ Does your job involve repetitive movements?

Repetitive tasks, apart from being psychologically problematic, can cause repetitive strain injury. Typing, for instance, can cause tenosynovitis, an inflammation of the sheaths within which the tendons to the fingers run. This causes pain, tenderness and swelling across the back of the wrist. And it's not just keyboard users who are at risk. Violinists, for example, must also be taught good technique, as synovitis can end a promising career. It's important to recognise these conditions very early, and do something about them as soon as possible. Rest is vital and the condition usually resolves with physiotherapy. In the longer term, changes must be made whether it's in the office or in a violinist's technique.

If repetitive tasks are a big part of your job, talk to someone about office ergonomics, take regular rests and, if possible, rotate these tasks with other jobs.

■ What's your work environment like?

Poor-quality air and dim or overbright light, together with loud or constant noise, can raise your stress levels and damage your health, as in 'sick building syndrome'. So how can you improve your occupational health? And what about wider issues of occupational health for people who don't work in office environments?

While working as a GP, I also served as an occupational health doctor for my local health authority, which meant that I was involved in looking after the health and safety of people in all sorts of different jobs in the hospital. I encountered a range of occupational problems caused by the widely differing working conditions experienced by plumbers, janitors, medical and nursing staff and office and admin workers. I found that many people fail to gauge the importance of occupational health issues; sometimes they don't see that their health is being affected, and miss out on chances to make often quite simple changes that would help them.

Some occupational health hazards are more obvious than others – if you work with radiation or dangerous chemicals you're more likely to be aware of occupational risks. Most people, however, work in an office of some sort, where occupational health issues are less likely to be taken quite so seriously. But the first step in improving your occupational health is to recognise that there are real risks and problems wherever you work, and to ask whether they could be affecting you.

Take another look at the list of ergonomics-related problems in the previous pages. Are you suffering from any of the symptoms described? Do any of your co-workers have similar problems? A tell-tale sign of 'sick building syndrome', for instance, is that while individual symptom patterns are vague and inconclusive, they are shared by several people working in the same place.

Practical ergonomics

The ideal working environment is rare, so how can you improve your environment, or, failing that, learn to cope with it to minimise the problems it may cause? Remember that this advice applies equally well to a variety of work environments – substitute machine, steering wheel, counter or cash till for workstation, depending on your job.

- **Work on your posture.** Bad posture is the number one culprit for back and neck problems that develop at work, and not just for white collar jobs. Whether you're a builder, electrician, nurse, lorry driver, chef, factory worker, teacher or landscape gardener, you need to pay careful attention to your seated and standing postures, and to how you bend over, lift, push or move things.

- **Sit comfortably.** Set up your workstation in the most ergonomic way possible. Ideally you should be able to reach everything you need from your seat without having to twist or stretch uncomfortably (if you can't reach something this way, get up to do it). Your keyboard should be squarely in front of you, at the right height to allow you to type with your arms at an angle of 70 to 90 degrees to your abdomen. Your screen or monitor should be within 30 degrees of your line of vision to prevent eye-strain.

- **Take a break**. Decent office chairs can be very expensive and are often not set up or used correctly anyway. Take care that your seating arrangements enable you to sit with good seat and back support. Even if you have the best seat possible, your body isn't designed for sitting around all day. The most obvious solution is to get up and walk around at frequent intervals – stretching your legs is also a good way to reduce the risk of deep vein thrombosis (DVT). The risk of DVT increases during any prolonged period of sitting and inactivity, not just on aeroplanes. One patient of mine had suffered a DVT after sitting for many hours, preparing his tax return. Truck or taxi drivers can also be at risk.

- **Do some stretching** – ideally, some simple back, arm and leg stretches when you get up from your workstation. If you don't think it'll go down well in the office, try and find a secluded spot to do your stretching. If it's not practical for you to be getting up regularly from your desk, do some seated stretching exercises.

  1. Sit up straight, arms straight down to the side, palms touching your chair. Gently, while pulling your tummy in, keeping shoulders square to the front, reach slowly to one side down towards the floor with your fingertips, stretching your side muscles. Allow your head to flop towards your shoulder to stretch your neck. Stretch progressively down each side. Do not stretch more than is comfortable for you.

  2. Sit up straight; raise elbows up and to the side. Try to move each elbow as far round to each side as possible, twisting your trunk and shoulders round, to rotate your spine.

3. Heels on the floor, raise your toes off the ground and hold for a count of five.

4. Lift each foot and rotate ankles up and down, and round in both directions.

5. Sit up straight and squeeze shoulder blades backwards, then forwards as far as possible. This can feel very relaxing and reduce tension.

6. Rotate wrists in both directions.

7. Put each leg out straight in turn, keeping your other leg bent and your back supported by your chair, raise toes and hold, then lift leg three times.

- **Get active**, even if only during your lunch break. If there's a gym or a pool near your office, you could break up the monotony of sitting in an uncomfortable position with some exercise that will get your circulation going, and make you stronger and more supple. If you've already got work-related problems such as back pain, obviously you'd need to take it easy at first. Later you could concentrate on exercises to strengthen your back. Even if you don't fancy spending your lunch break working out, make sure you get out of the office and stretch your legs outside. Don't sit at your desk for lunch!

- **Give your eyes a break**, which will help you avoid eyestrain and headaches. Apart from setting up your workstation properly, make sure that your working area, your screen and keyboard are well lit – with indirect natural light if possible. If you can't see them properly you may be straining forward or down without realising it. Try to cultivate the habit of looking away from the screen, gazing into the distance and closing your eyes for a few seconds at frequent intervals. If you wear glasses or lenses, make sure you get your prescription checked. (Tell your optician you use a VDU.)

- **Get a better keyboard**, particularly if you already have a repetitive strain problem. Ergonomic keyboards are now widely available, and easily recognised by their split, curved or angled keypads. For the really badly affected, there are all sorts of clever input devices, from a stenographer's-style chord keypad to completely hands-free voice recognition software. Do check out new options as they become available.

- **Keep the noise down.** A noisy working environment isn't just more stressful, it can actually cause short and long-term damage to your hearing – such as a degree of hearing loss and tinnitus. I'm not only talking about the obviously noisy jobs, like machine operator or roadie for a band, but also white collar professions such as stockbroking. Workstation screens, ear plugs or defenders are one option. Talk to your employer (see below), but if you're self-employed be sure to take equal care of yourself.

When to make a fuss – and seek help

One obvious problem with taking steps to improve your working environment is that, because ergonomics and similar issues aren't taken very seriously in many jobs, or may not seem obvious, your boss may not seem to be very sympathetic. But if you think your work conditions are affecting you, you must make this very clear to your employer or occupational health department. In the UK, employers are legally required to follow Health and Safety Executive (HSE) guidelines, which are actually very comprehensive and, if followed, assure a reasonable working environment. HSE guidelines cover everything from temperature and lighting to noise levels and exposure to toxic fumes. The first place I send self-employed patients who are worried about occupational health issues (for example, craft activities, woodturning and home photography labs) is to have a look at the HSE guidelines for their profession from government websites, so your employers will be doing the same. Do talk to your boss and the human resources manager about it.

If you've developed problems as a result of poor ergonomics, or if your job puts you 'in harm's way', think about seeking help from your doctor, a naturopath, or a specialist such as an osteopath or physiotherapist. There are specialist physiotherapists for some professions – such as musicians – and they are especially important early in a person's career when it is essential to develop good postural and ergonomic habits.

CHAPTER 14

Patient power

M any aspects of physical health clearly cannot be properly evaluated at home or by looking in the mirror – they must be investigated with tests or screens that can only be done by or through your doctor. Screening is an important part of any total health programme, but very few people understand just how important it is, and most do not know which types of test they should be having and when. The questions below are intended to help you determine whether any particular types of screening are indicated for you personally. I believe you should be proactive about your health – and knowing the options available to you are an important part of that.

I'd also like to encourage you to be assertive about your health care. It's a two-way street. If you have questions, do ask them, and ensure that you feel they have been answered to your satisfaction.

SCREENING TESTS YOU COULD NEED

- In the last two years, have you had any of the following screenings? Blood pressure check; blood analysis, including screening for anaemia, cholesterol levels and fasting blood sugar; urine test; lung function test; resting electrocardiogram; chest X-ray; vision and glaucoma testing; hearing test; dental check-up; and, for the

---

over-fifties, faecal occult blood screening and consideration of colonoscopy. For those over 40 with a family history of glaucoma, have you been screened for this (screening should by yearly)? If you have a family history of bowel cancer or polyps, have you had a colonoscopy?

- Do you suffer from pain in your abdomen from heartburn or acid reflux?

- Do you suffer from recurrent urinary tract infections?

- Do you suffer from impotence or urinary problems, or, if a woman, from dyspareunia (painful intercourse), vaginal dryness or arousal problems?

- Do you have an apple or pear-shaped figure?

- Do you suffer from any of the following symptoms? Chest pain; palpitations; shortness of breath; pain in the arms, lower back or down the sides.

- Do you ever get light-headed or faint?

- Do you suffer from coldness of the extremities or pain in the calves on walking?

- Do you suffer from shortness of breath, wheezing and noisy breathing?

- Have you suffered from an episode of jaundice or intense pain in the abdomen and back?

- Do you suffer from frequent attacks of colds, flu or herpes; chronic infections; swollen glands?

- Do you have any new moles, or existing moles that have changed shape, size or colour, become rough or irregular, started bleeding or itching?

- Do you feel that it's up to your doctor to cure you when you get ill?

- Do you think that your doctor won't listen to your complaints, or that a visit to the surgery is likely to be a waste of time?

- Are you afraid of what you might discover if you go and see the doctor?

- Are you happy with your current GP?

- Do you research your health problems and possible treatment options?

- Do you believe that 'doctor knows best'?

- Do you ever challenge or question your doctor? Would you feel confident about doing so?

- Do you pay attention to your 'inner doctor' – the messages coming from your own body; the intuitions about what you need and don't need?

■ What types of screening have you undergone in the last two years?

I consider the following tests for all my patients.

- **Blood pressure check** to screen for hypertension (high blood pressure), risk factors for stroke and cardiovascular disease. Normal blood pressure for adults is ideally not higher than 140/80. However, if you have diabetes, kidney disease, or established heart disease, your target is 130/80 or lower.

- **Blood analysis.** A comprehensive blood analysis includes a 'full blood count', screening for anaemia and other blood abnormalities, cholesterol levels with a breakdown of blood fats (levels of fats after fasting – known as a 'full fasting lipid profile') and fasting blood sugar (levels of glucose in your blood after fasting). A 'biochemistry profile' screens for problems such as abnormal function of the liver (signs of drinking excess alcohol, kidney problems and gout); I would also consider screening for nutritional deficiencies (such as of iron or vitamin B12). These basic screening tests provide alerts on diabetes or heart disease risk factors and to liver or kidney problems, blood disorders and gout.

- **Urine reagent stick tests** check for protein and glucose sugar in the blood in order to screen for diabetes, kidney disease, urinary tract infection and risk factors for kidney stones.

- **A urine culture test** may confirm urinary tract infection.

- **Lung function tests** check the function and capacity of the lungs. The simplest test is called a 'peak flow' in which a doctor asks the patient to blow out rapidly into a small meter. Further tests include detailed lung function tests or spirometry, which give more information about lung capacity and function. Lung tests screen for asthma, bronchitis or emphysema, and are also a good measure of general fitness, and therefore of risk factors for respiratory disease.

- **Resting electrocardiograms** record your heart rate and rhythm. They screen for arrhythmia (abnormal rhythm), an indicator of cardiovascular problems.

- **Chest X-rays** can be suitable for some patients. These look for signs of tuberculosis (TB), lung cancer, emphysema and other respiratory diseases such as chronic bronchitis or sarcoid (a granulomatous condition).

- **Vision screening** includes tests of visual acuity to check your focus and to assess whether you may be short or long-sighted, and whether you need glasses and screening for glaucoma. Glaucoma is a surprisingly common disorder where excess fluid builds up in the eye, causing an increase in pressure. It can cause blindness if left untreated, but is easily controlled if detected. As a general rule, you should have your vision tested to check your prescription at least every two years – and more frequently if you have a family history of glaucoma or you are advised to do so. Examination of the eyes also provides useful information about diabetic or hypertensive complications, as both these conditions cause visible changes in blood vessels at the back of the eyes.

- **Hearing tests** become more important with age. Hearing impairment can affect your social life and general level of engagement with the world around you, but many people don't even realise the extent of their hearing deficit. People who have been exposed to loud sounds or noise pollution on a regular basis, such as factory workers or heavy metal fans, should take care to get their hearing assessed.

- **Dental check-up.** You should have one every six months, to check your teeth, assess gum health and screen for oral cancers. It is important that dentures fit properly. Your dentist will also check for misalignments of the teeth (known as malocclusions), which can give rise to headaches.

- **Faecal occult blood screening** is a test checking for blood in the stool – a warning sign for bowel cancer. It's advisable for people over 50, or anyone with risk factors such as irregular bowel habit or a family history of either bowel polyps or cancer. Ask your relatives about this; otherwise you may not find out.

- **Colonoscopy.** A direct inspection of the colon with an endoscope (a tiny camera on a flexible rod using fibre-optic technology) to check for polyps (growths in the bowel), inflammatory bowel disorders and bowel cancer. Again, in many countries, this is recommended routinely for people over 50 or anyone with risk factors.

What about tests for men?

Several important types of screening are gender-specific, which is why most clinics offer versions of a 'well-man' or 'well-woman' screen. For male patients I advise the following screening tests, in addition to the 'unisex' ones listed above:

- **Testicular examination** (and instruction in self-examination). Testicular cancer is a major threat to men of all ages and in very many cases affects men under 40, but public awareness of the condition, and more importantly of how to check for it, is worryingly poor. Just as women should be aware of changes in their breasts such as lumps, pain or nipple discharge, and should report them, so men need to make testicular self-examination a regular habit. A doctor can show you how this is done while doing this screen.

When boys are growing up it is useful to tell them that their 'balls' should both feel the same as usual and that they should tell their parent or doctor about any changes. Certainly my two sons are aware of this.

CHECKING YOUR TESTICLES

You need to know what's normal for you. It can be perfectly normal to have one testicle a little larger or higher than the other. But they should both be about the same size and weight. Feel each testicle and roll it gently between your thumb and fingers. It should feel smooth. You will feel a soft, tender structure (the epididymis) towards the back of each testicle. Report any changes whatsoever and any pain or tenderness. Warning signs of testicular cancer are often obvious and easy to find. Watch out for one or more of the following:

- A hard lump on the surface of the testicle

- A swelling or enlargement

- An increase in firmness

- Pain or discomfort

- An unusual difference between one testicle and the other

- A heavy or dragging feeling in the groin, or a dull ache in the lower stomach or groin

- Any of these changes should be reported to your GP without delay. Even though they may be due to other causes, they need to be investigated.

- **Prostate-specific antigen testing.** Elevated levels in the blood of a protein known as prostate-specific antigen may act as a marker for potential prostate problems. Although a raised level may have a variety of causes, this information can be very useful in planning whether further investigations to detect prostate conditions, including cancer, are necessary.

Testing should be accompanied by a discussion of any family history of prostate cancer and the presence of symptoms of prostate disorder.

What about tests for women?

Important screens that I recommend to my female patients are:

- **Blood test for rubella** (aka 'German measles'), for women of childbearing age. Contracting rubella during pregnancy can have very serious consequences for the foetus, so it's advisable to get screened to see if you are already immune to the disease (through earlier infection or inoculation), or whether you might be vulnerable. A simple blood test can reveal whether you carry antibodies to the virus – if you are not immune you can discuss vaccination with your doctor.

- **Pelvic examination** – a manual internal examination carried out by a doctor and possibly pelvic ultrasound examinations, using either a trans-abdominal or trans-vaginal probe. Ultrasound examination provides images of the pelvic organs to check the size and shape of the uterus and ovaries, and will identify ovarian cysts and other masses or fibroids. Trans-vaginal ultrasound is a relatively new technique where the ultrasound probe is inserted into the vagina rather than simply passed over the outside of the abdomen. It provides clearer pictures of the pelvic organs because the probe gets closer and the image is less obscured by the abdominal wall, fatty tissue or gas in the intestines.

- **Ovarian cancer screening** should be considered for those with a family history of the disease. This involves both trans-vaginal ultrasound using a technique to reveal abnormal blood flow and tumour-marker studies (a blood test known as Ca^{125} screening) to check for the presence of proteins that can indicate that a tumour may be developing. Available screening may reveal 'false positives', which can be anxiety-provoking, but the aim is early detection of borderline changes before a cancer has developed and progressed. Early diagnosis will improve outcome. For women considered to be at great risk, screening should be considered by a gynaecologist on an annual basis. Your GP should be able to advise you about specialist centres that are researching this type of screening.

- **Breast examination** (and instruction in self-examination) to check for cysts or lumps. Extensive education programmes about the dangers of breast cancer have raised public awareness, but many women still don't check their breasts to get used to how they normally feel and change through a menstrual cycle. Again, early diagnosis leads to better outcomes for women with breast cancer.

- **Mammogram** with breast ultrasound. If you have a family history of breast cancer or are otherwise at high risk, discuss with your doctor whether you should start having mammograms at a younger age than is normally required.

- **Cervical (or pap) smear,** to check for abnormalities in cervical cells which may indicate cervical cancer or pre-cancerous changes..

BREAST AWARENESS

Being breast aware is simple to do and it doesn't mean following a strict or complicated routine. It just means knowing what your breasts look and feel like normally. Do this in any way that makes you feel most comfortable – in the bath, shower, when dressing, standing up or lying down.

If you find anything unusual or are worried then contact your GP as soon as possible. Lumps are not the only things to watch out for, so look out for the following:

- A lumpy area or thickening of the breast that doesn't disappear after your period

- A change in the size or shape of the breast

- A change in the skin of the breast such as dimpling or puckering

- A change in the nipple – in appearance or direction, or any blood-stained or other discharge

- Breast pain that doesn't resolve after your period

If you have any of these symptoms, contact your GP as soon as possible. You should be referred on an urgent basis to a specialist breast clinic if your GP is concerned.

■ Do you suffer from pain in your abdomen from heart-burn or acid reflux?

This, and the following questions, are signs and symptoms that indicate you should consult your GP. Do not ignore any symptoms.

If you are experiencing pain in the abdomen, is it in the lower or upper abdomen? Lower abdominal pain is more likely to be associated with bowel disorders or gynaecological problems in women. Upper abdominal pain tends to be associated with disorders of the stomach, liver, gallbladder, pancreas and bowel. Nevertheless. there are overlaps and these organs lie close to each other, so all possible diagnoses should be considered.

The nature of the pain can help narrow the diagnosis – is it constant, or does it come and go, as with colic? (Pain from gallstones or kidney stones is characteristically 'colicky', as is some bowel pain.) Are there other symptoms alongside your pain? For example, acid reflux with upper abdominal pain, or constipation with lower abdominal pain? If you have noticed any rectal bleeding or symptoms that are persistent or accompanied by unexpected weight loss, they require urgent medical investigation, and you may be referred for an endoscopy – an internal inspection of the gut with a flexible fibre-optic instrument.

A gastroscopy is a fibre-optic examination down through the mouth and oesophagus into the stomach and duodenum to identify areas of inflammation or ulceration.

A colonoscopy is an examination of the inside and lining of the large bowel (colon) to reveal polyps, diverticular disease, inflammation or tumour.

You may choose to be sedated for these examinations.

Samples of tissue (biopsies) can also be taken during endoscopic examination for laboratory (histological) examination. Polyps (protrusions from the bowel wall) will be checked for signs of malignancy. Inflammatory changes seen in ulcerative colitis or Crohn's disease can also be confirmed, and diverticular disease (involving small pouches in the bowel which can become inflamed) identified.

NICK OF TIME

A 45-year-old student called Annie came to see me complaining of the classic symptoms of irritable bowel syndrome (IBS) – alternating constipation and diarrhoea, bloating and wind, and sometimes slimy bowel movements. She was under a lot of stress because of exams, and assumed that this was making her IBS worse – so bad, in fact, that she was losing weight.

Although Annie had no family history of bowel cancer, I was concerned that her symptoms might indicate something more serious, and also that she had been diagnosed with IBS without any gastroenterological investigations. As I explained to her, IBS should be considered a 'diagnosis of exclusion' – in other words, it's what you label the disorder when you can't find any other physical cause for the symptoms. Before you can make a diagnosis of IBS, therefore, you need to have considered and excluded all the other possible causes. The older the patient, the more likely it is that there may be underlying pathology, so the greater the need to investigate.

My suspicions proved to be well founded. A colonoscopy exam showed the presence of multiple polyps, which can become malignant and develop into bowel cancer. Her polyps were removed and were happily benign but she is at increased risk of bowel cancer and so will undergo colonoscopy every few years or so as advised by her surgeon. As polyps can affect families I advised her to tell her sister in the US. She too was found to have bowel polyps and will also remain under surveillance by colonoscopy to prevent bowel cancer.

Unfortunately, I've seen many other cases where patients were treated for IBS without being properly diagnosed, allowing bowel cancers to develop too far to be easily treated. But remember doctors can only help if people take their concerns to them.

■ Do you suffer from recurrent urinary tract infections?

For women, recurrent urinary tract infections (UTIs) can be symptomatic of sexually transmitted infections (STIs), inflammation or abnormalities of the urinary tract, diabetes or other causes of poor immune function. You will need urine and blood tests, and for recurrent infections your doctor may refer you to a urologist, who deals with kidney and bladder problems, or a gynaecologist. For men, UTIs can also indicate STI problems, abnormalities of the urinary tract or prostatitis – and screening will be needed.

PROTECT YOUR URINARY TRACT

1. Wipe your bottom from front to back if you're a woman to avoid pulling germs up from the anus to the urethra. In a woman, the urethra is very short and bacteria will enter the bladder very easily.

2. Drink plenty of water every day (2 litres or so) to ensure you empty your bladder regularly. This will prevent any build-up of stray bacteria from the bowel. Most urinary tract infections are caused by bowel bacteria.

3. Consider taking cranberry juice or powder. It inhibits bacterial growth, but you may need to drink it daily, not just during an attack.

4. As soon as possible after the start of an attack, take a urine sample (taken in 'mid-stream') to your doctor for analysis. Urinary tract infections can travel up to the kidneys and antibiotics may be necessary. Also, drink frequent cups of warm water with the remedy potassium citrate mixture, called Mist Pot Cit (available from chemists) to reduce painful acidity in the bladder. After a course of antibiotics, take probiotic acidophilus capsules for a week or so to restore healthy gut flora.

5. If you suffer from recurrent UTIs, your GP will need to rule out kidney problems and vaginal infections.

■ Are you having sexual problems?

Sexual dysfunction can stem from a variety of medical and emotional roots. Don't feel embarrassed that you're having problems in this area: speak with your doctor or practice nurse at the outset. Some problems are to do with medication (for depression or raised blood pressure, for example), stress and overwork, hormonal issues (around menopause) or diabetes. Many people develop 'performance anxiety', making the problem worse. But with a sensitive approach, you can alleviate or eradicate the problem. Your doctor will consider some medical investigations, and a review of medication. You may benefit from some counselling.

MEDICAL BASIS OF SEXUAL PROBLEMS

He . . .

- **Can't get an erection**. It can happen to anyone, and, having happened once or twice, the fear of a recurrence can make it even more likely. However, impotence can also be a sign of narrowing arteries (causing heart disease), diabetes or a side effect of some medication, so talk to your GP.

- **Has a curvature to his penis**. Curvature can be caused by Peyronie's disease, in which fibrous plaques form in the shaft of the penis. It's quite rare – only affecting one or two in a hundred men – but see your GP to discuss treatment. He may refer you to a specialist for further discussion.

- **Can't ejaculate**. Delayed ejaculation can be a sign of diabetes, nerve damage or prostate disease. Some medicines can also affect ejaculation, as can drinking too heavily.

She . . .

- **Finds sex painful**. Intercourse should not be painful and if it becomes so, either on penetration or during deep intercourse, a cause must be found. Very deep penetration in the 'doggy' position may cause discomfort, but the 'missionary' position should not. Watch out for any

---

unusual discharge or bleeding – which could be a sign of infection and can also cause sex to be painful. Other underlying causes that may need to be ruled out include disease of the cervix, ovarian cysts or tumour, endometriosis (where uterine lining is scattered outside of the uterus and bleeds, causing cysts and pain) and bowel disorders.

- **Feels 'too dry'.** Cigarettes, allergy medicines, and the Pill can all affect your lubrication, but the most common cause is the menopause, when oestrogen levels decline. Aloe vera and yam creams can help, but talk to your GP, who may request swabs or blood tests to check hormone levels.

- **Doesn't climax as she used to.** Weaker orgasms, like stress incontinence, may be a sign that you need to strengthen your pelvic floor muscles. While sitting, tighten your urethra, vagina and anus together as hard as you can. Aim to squeeze for 10 seconds (at first you may only manage 2 to 3 seconds. Relax for 10 seconds and then repeat the exercise 10 times in all. Do this three times a day. If you have difficulty locating the muscle and can't feel a squeezing sensation, your doctor may refer you to a physiotherapist for help. Another useful exercise is to do 10 short, sharp squeezes three times a day. Any woman who does not have orgasms, or suffers tightness of the vagina caused by spasm of vaginal muscles during attempted intercourse, should see her GP, who can offer a referral to a gynaecologist, and/or psychosexual counselling.

■ Do you have an apple or pear-shaped figure?

A pear-shaped figure is the body type where your hips are broad compared to your waist, and may put you at lower risk of cardiovascular problems. But an apple-shaped figure, where you are big around the waist compared to your hips, is considered a relatively higher risk factor for cardiovascular disease.

There are two ways you can work out whether you are carrying an unhealthy amount of fat.

The hip/waist ratio reflects the distribution of fat on the body, and is therefore the best way to tell if someone is an apple or a pear. To work out your own hip/waist ratio, simply divide your waist measurement by your hip measurement. Ideally, women should have a waist-to-hip ratio of 0.8 or less. Men should ideally have a waist-to-hip ratio of 0.95 or less. For example, take Belinda, whose measurements are waist, 91 cm and hips, 101 cm. She would calculate 91 divided by 101, which gives her a waist-to-hip ratio of 0.9, which is higher than the ideal figure.

If your hip/waist ratio is not desirable, then it would be a good idea to see your doctor to discuss your eating patterns and level of physical activity.

Your body mass index or BMI is a measure of your weight in proportion to your height and is used to determine whether that proportion is healthy or not. It's easy to work out: divide your weight in kilos by your height in metres squared. For example, if you weight 60kg and are 1.65 m tall then: 60kg divided by [1.65 x 1.65 = 2.72] = 22.03. A BMI of 20 to 24.9 is healthy, 25 to 29.9 is overweight, and 30 or above is obese. And unfortunately, a growing number of people in the West – even those who 'carry their weight well' – are obese.

■ Do you suffer from cardiovascular-related symptoms?

Palpitations, shortness of breath on exertion and chest pain on exertion – maybe spreading to the left arm or jaw – indicate cardiovascular problems, and need to be thoroughly checked by a doctor using electrocardiogram and other tests. Chest pain relieved by rest is particularly suggestive of angina, a condition in which the coronary vessels allow inadequate blood to the heart muscle.

■ Do you ever get light-headed or faint?

Light-headedness or fainting may indicate problems with blood pressure (get your pressure checked), or with blood sugar. Light-headedness is also more likely in someone who is anaemic or prone to palpitations or a disturbed heart rhythm, and all these things should be tested.

▦ Do you suffer from cold feet or cramps in your calves when walking?

These may indicate a blockage or narrowing of the arteries (intermittent claudication), possibly caused by atherosclerosis or peripheral vascular disease with subsequent reduction of blood flow to the legs. Anyone with these symptoms should always be checked out by a vascular surgeon (your GP can refer you).

▦ Do you suffer from shortness of breath, wheezing and noisy breathing?

These respiratory symptoms may suggest asthma, bronchitis or emphysema, or maybe a cardiac issue. A doctor might investigate further with lung function tests, a chest X-ray and blood tests. Anaemia can also cause shortness of breath.

▦ Do you suffer from attacks of intermittent pain in the upper abdomen, or jaundice, heartburn or acid reflux?

Upper abdominal pain can be caused by disorders of the liver, gallbladder, stomach or pancreas. Liver or gallbladder problems may cause jaundice (yellowing of the whites of the eyes, and the skin), and needs urgent investigation. Gallstones are a common cause. Dyspepsia (heartburn) and acid reflux may indicate inflammation or ulceration. Do not ignore this or persist in taking 'over the counter' antacids. Your doctor will arrange tests for a bacterium called *Helicobacter pylori* that can promote such problems. A gastroscopy may also be ordered.

▦ Are you prone to getting colds, flu or herpes attacks; chronic infections; swollen glands?

Your resistance to colds, flu and other ailments is a good barometer of how well your health reserves are doing. The stronger your reserves, the quicker you'll be able to overcome infections and regain your natural balance – and the more resistant your system will be to the disturbances of equilibrium that cause ill health. If you get ill a lot, however, it's a clear sign that your reserves are failing, probably because something is draining them. That 'something' is more than likely to do with your diet or your environment, but it may not be anything specific. Illnesses, especially common ones likes colds and flu, can be the result of a gradual build-up of problems stretching the capacity of your system to breaking point. The 'exciting cause', the factor that appears to be responsible for the illness, is usually simply the final trigger that tips your system's equilibrium over the threshold. So a bout of flu is not simply the result of infection with a flu virus; the virus may only be the exciting cause, and follow a series of stresses affecting your biochemical health.

If your resitance to this kind of illness is low, this can indicate problems with the immune system – initial investigation involves blood tests.

■ Have you noticed any changes in your moles?

Changes in shape, size or colour, roughness or irregularity, and bleeding in moles can be warning signs that a previously benign mole is malignant or undergoing a malignant change. Do not delay in dealing with this. It's important to ask your doctor to look at any new or changed moles immediately, and, if necessary, you will be referred to a dermatologist for urgent assessment and appropriate management. The number of cases of malignant melanoma is escalating, and early diagnosis is absolutely essential for successful treatment.

Taking charge of your health

Your answers to the previous questions may have highlighted areas of concern in the physical corner of your triangle of health. In order to address these concerns you will need your doctor's help and advice – to perform the tests and screens described above, to help you understand what the results mean and to decide what to do next.

So your relationship with your doctor is vital to your goal of reaching and maintaining a state of total health. That relationship, however, is only part of your overall approach to healthcare. The following questions will help you to assess whether you have the right approach, and whether you are getting the most out of your relationship with your doctor.

■ Do you feel that it's up to your doctor to cure you?

As I said early on in this book, during all my years in NHS general practice I have found that many of my patients felt that their health was my problem. They would turn up at the surgery, present their symptoms and wait for me to prescribe some sort of medication or treatment that would cure them.

By taking a passive role in their own healthcare, they had ceased to be responsible for their own wellbeing. All the power in the doctor-patient relationship was on one side only, a set-up that breeds dependence and a sense of helplessness. By contrast, patients who are actively involved, and who take charge of their own health, tend to have much better outcomes. They are more likely to take better care of themselves, follow treatment regimes more faithfully, adopt and maintain lifestyle changes and develop a more positive outlook (the benefits of a real doctor-patient partnership).

You may recognise that you are the passive type, or that you rarely follow the advice you're given. But it is possible to make your internal voice more positive. Numerous patients come to me with problems that are not life-threatening, saying, 'I've been to so many doctors and I'm still stuck with this chronic problem.' Unfortunately, they may remain stuck with the problem until they view their healthcare as teamwork, and ask, 'What can I do to improve the chances of successful treatment?'

■ Do you think that your doctor won't listen to your complaints, or that a visit to the surgery is likely to be a waste of time?

Your GP's surgery is often your gateway to all the other medical services you need, so it's important to feel that your doctor is listening to you, and taking your problem seriously. Only by getting your message across will you get the follow-up tests or referral to a specialist you require. Examine your assumptions. If you approach healthcare with negative expectations, you are more likely to have a negative outcome. If you are positive, you are more likely to get the most out of the healthcare services.

■ Are you afraid of what you might discover if you go and see your doctor?

Anxieties like this are natural and understandable, and common among 'the worried well'. You need to overcome your fear – don't let it prevent you from getting important tests or treatment. Diagnosing a condition early means you can do something about it. Not knowing means you may or may not have it – but if you do, the wait till you finally decide to go to the doctor means treatment may well become far more complicated, with less prospect of a good outcome.

■ Are you happy with your current GP?

Finding a physician who can be a good partner in your healthcare is vital. As leading health writer Christiane Northrup puts it, 'The effect of working with a healer you trust and believe in is *physical*, as much a part of your healing as the mode of treatment you actually choose.' You have the right to change your doctor if you want to and you can do this at any time without having to give a reason. You should feel comfortable with your doctor and confident in him or her.

■ Do you research your health problems and possible treatment options?

The more you know about your condition and the treatment options available, the more choices will be open to you and the more confident you can be about making them. Read about and research both general and specific health issues.

■ Do you believe that 'doctor knows best'?

In too many clinics and surgeries, patients are expected and expect to confine themselves to answering the doctor's questions and following the doctor's prescription. The implicit message is that 'doctor knows best' and that you should consent to examination and/or treatment without too many questions. I've heard many patients say that they are worried that they may upset their doctor if they ask questions or talk about things they've learned through their own research. You should feel comfortable raising any issue with your GP.

■ Do you ever challenge or question your doctor?

If you're unsure about something your doctor has said or done, and you're worried that you lack confidence or might feel intimidated when confronting them, take a friend with you to act as a surrogate voice. Any consultation may leave you with questions as well as answers. Don't be afraid to go back for clarification.

'I'M TOO DEPENDENT ON MEDICATION'

Matt, an accountant in his forties, came to see me about long-standing symptoms that had been attributed to an irritable bowel. Specialist investigation had not been able to find any underlying disease that might be causing the symptoms and all that doctors had been able to prescribe were laxatives and anti-spasmodic drugs to control the symptoms. By the time Matt arrived in my office he had, amazingly, been taking the same drugs for over 20 years, in slowly but steadily increasing doses.

When I pressed him, he admitted that he wasn't happy with the situation, but what could he do? His doctors had told him there was nothing else they could do, that there was no serious underlying illness, and that he should take the medication if he wanted to avoid the worst symptoms. It was apparent to me that his approach to his healthcare was tied in with his approach to the rest of life. He was very devoted to his family and wanted to provide well for them. He worked long hours, and was continually anxious that he wasn't doing enough, although he was, by most people's standards, very successful. It seemed to me that he had fallen into a deeply ingrained pattern of 'self-sacrifice'. He had a tendency always to put himself and his own needs last, and could never find time to exercise or to pay much attention on his diet.

Through a good deal of patience and coaxing I was able to get Matt to talk about what he really wanted in terms of treatment. His first priority was to reduce his dependence on his medication, which he had begun to feel was making things worse, not better. Although there was no evidence that this was actually the case, I thought that it was the principle that was more important, and encouraged him to think about alternative forms of treatment that he might prefer.

Together we worked out a treatment plan that involved making small but practical lifestyle changes on a day-by-day basis. He started exercising regularly, improved his diet through the introduction of vegetable juicing and worked on his bowel habits by learning to take his time when visiting the lavatory and practising relaxation techniques while there. Gradually he developed a regular, daily bowel habit, and weaned himself off his 20-year-long prescription. Matt's problems went deeper than just irregular bowel habits, however, so I introduced him to the counselling process and a course of relaxation techniques and breathing exercises. These helped him open the door to making the changes outlined above, and greatly enhanced his peace of mind.

Matt's case again illustrates the importance of addressing all three corners of the triangle of health – physical, biochemical and psychological. Crucially, he learned to take charge of his own healthcare process instead of simply following the advice of doctors without question. The benefits for him have extended far beyond the relief of his IBS symptoms.

■ Do you pay attention to your 'inner doctor'?

Your inner 'guidance system' – the messages coming from your own body – can be a powerful force, but this phenomenon is traditionally undervalued by conventional medicine. Losing touch with it is disempowering, and this disempowerment can have physical consequences.

If something doesn't feel right to you, voice your concerns. Despite what many doctors might say, you are probably the best judge of your body. Don't be afraid to disagree with a doctor or ask for a second opinion, and if there's a real conflict between what you feel inside and what your caregiver says, explain your concerns and try to reach an agreement. Remember – remain fully involved in your own healthcare.

PATIENT POWER

- Believe in patient power

- It is also down to you to know when to ask for further help. If you have a concern about your health you must voice it

- Do not accept second best. Patients who take an active interest in their own health generally respond more successfully to treatment

---

PART **4**

Psychological Health

CHAPTER 15

Remembrance of things past

I f you're fit and eating well, you're laying the best foundations for mental as well as physical health. And it works the other way too: your psychological health affects your overall state of health. Harking back to your health triangle, remember – your reserves of mental energy and resilience are as important as your nutritional and physical reserves.

It's fortunate that this fact is slowly filtering through to conventional medicine. There is now a whole area of research, psychoneuroimmunology, which studies how mental states, particularly stress, may influence the immune system by boosting or suppressing its activity. Doctors and hospitals are increasingly aware that happier patients respond better to treatment, recover quicker and relapse less than people who are anxious or depressed, and now make more effort to match physical care with mental and spiritual care – for example, by providing light airy spaces with plants, where patients can sit and watch the world go by. Both environment, and good information, dissipate anxiety. I certainly found myself feeling very isolated when I was stuck in a side room on my own in hospital 10 years ago – and felt much better when I could get into some sunshine and feel less institutionalised.

It's important to keep this close interaction between mind and body in focus when you're assessing aspects of your own inner life. Certainly, I see this interconnectedness every day in my practice.

I want you to look back at your life history and think about the major influences and events that shaped your personality and path through life. Then I will ask you to look at your life as it is today and think about your lifestyle, responsibilities and relationships. This exercise should help you make an honest appraisal of your state of mind and gain insight into issues that might be holding you back from achieving mental equilibrium – in other words, 'peace of mind'.

Many of my patients come to see me because they're suffering from chronic ailments that conventional treatments have failed to cure. When they also complain that they feel their lives are stuck in a rut, it doesn't take a genius to see how emotional states might affect a person's physical condition. Dealing with emotional issues and stress requires the will to make changes, and sometimes professional support. It is important to develop insight into the roots of those problems. This is precisely why I feel that it's so important to take a life history alongside a medical history.

Life stages – and the Potted Life History

A conventional GP builds up a picture of his or her patient's background over the course of repeated visits which – if you're lucky enough to have a long-term relationship with your doctor – may span many years. In my naturopathic practice I have to try to achieve something similar in less than an hour during an initial consultation. The method I use is what I call the 'Potted Life History' approach, and basically involves finding out about the highlights and turning points in my patient's childhood, adolescence and adult life. These influences tell me a lot about where my patients are coming from. Our discussion also helps them to see how their characters and outlook may have influenced. Covering so much ground in such a short space of time is an essential part of my first consultation (which is always a fact-finding mission) and helps me put a person and their concerns 'into context'. It is a good starting point from which patients can identify key areas they may need to work on. Most people are happy to talk about themselves – especially to a sympathetic listener. The naturopathic approach very much utilises this essential 'art' of medicine, which I firmly believe should be woven back into conventional consulting skills.

Here I'm going to ask you to be your own sympathetic listener. It may sound self-indulgent, but it is a very therapeutic process, and, to make it work, it's vital to register how *you* felt about the various issues – not how they made your mother, father, siblings or partner feel.

Start by dividing your life into stages. Psychological development is a process that continues throughout life. Even as we move on to new concerns and challenges, unresolved issues from the past can still haunt us and failure to deal with them adequately can result in psychological 'baggage' or unfinished business that weighs us down. I tend to use the following life stages:

- Before birth
- Babyhood
- Toddler
- Preschool
- Childhood
- Puberty, adolescence, the teens
- Young adulthood
- Mature adult
- Middle age – 'prime years'
- Retiree
- Older age

Birth to preschool

Very few people can remember their lives before the age of around four. No one is exactly sure why this is, but psychologists call it 'infantile amnesia'. Whether or not you can consciously recall events from your early infancy, they may have made an impact on your developing personality, especially if they were particularly significant or momentous. How secure you felt as a young child may also influence later development. I clearly remember falling backwards down the stairs as a two-year-old struggling to take off my coat! It has left me with a distinct fear of heights and I did

not relish being taken on cliff-top walks by my husband on our honey-
moon!

More seriously, things like the death of a parent or sibling or an abrupt
and extreme change in your environment can cause problems in later life,
and the psychological consequences may feed into ill health.

Childhood

Your childhood years have had a very real impact on the adult you turned
out to be. During this time, the ebbs, flows, trials and tribulations within a
family powerfully affect a child's development, so we'll look at families
closely here.

The family environment   The family group – whatever its make-up, conventional or not — is the most important influence on childhood development, and, by extension, on the development of your adult personality. It's
the first social environment you encounter, and the place where you learn to
interact with other people, develop and express desires and goals and pursue and negotiate their fulfilment or deal with disappointments. The psychologist Erik Erikson (1902–1994), who described crises, or hurdles to be
overcome in our personal development, said that childhood involves developing initiative, which is in conflict with guilt over childish instincts and
fantasies. The crisis for the child is to resolve the conflict between initiative
and guilt. The lessons you learn in the family help you to cope with the wider
world. When you move into new environments, such as the classroom or
playground, you try to apply the skills and tactics that you developed in the
family environment.

Family geneagram   I ask my patients to tell me a little about their family,
and in particular to talk about who was an important influence or an especially close relative. This influence may be positive or negative. Lily was a well-
balanced young woman of about 26 who came to me about niggling health
problems. Her potted history revealed she'd had terrible relations with her
mother in the past. She'd always found it hard to meet her mother's high
expectations of her – and this came to a crunch when, taking against one of
Lily's boyfriends, her mother had Lily's dog put down as a punishment!

Amazingly, Lily had managed to pick herself up and carry on with her life. She still regularly visited her mother (who, incidentally, had never apologised for her horrible act), but she would never be able to forgive her. Lily was, as I've said, very well balanced and in spite of her relationship with her mother, she was quite healthy and able to lead a successful life.

Others are not so lucky. Unable to stand up for his own creative urges, Nigel toed the family line and tried to please his parents by becoming an accountant instead of an artist. As he lived what he felt was a 'grey' life, his stifled personality manifested as chronic listlessness and general malaise, and he needed my help to uncover what was going on, and revive his creative instinct.

In one school of psychotherapy, this kind of information is used to draw up a 'family geneagram'. This is a sort of family tree that notes not just births, deaths and marriages, but also any significant events in the family. These events typically include divorce, early deaths, serious accidents and significant physical or mental illnesses, and they tend to have great influence on family patterns.

In the diagram opposite, Jane's family geneagram reveals a history of depression and alcohol abuse. Rather than blaming herself, or wondering where she went wrong, Jane is now able to recognise that she is part of a family pattern. She can see that there may have been factors in her environment that contributed towards her developing these problems. With this knowledge, she will be able to deal with her depression and alcohol abuse with more insight and less blame.

Birth order To shift focus from you to your family in general, let's look at birth order. Your place in the family environment is partly determined by this – whether you were a first, middle or last child, an only child or perhaps the only boy among girls or vice versa. As a first-born child you would have had a particular relationship with your parents; if you were a later child your arrival would have changed the relationship between your older sibling(s) and your parents, and this may have affected your own relationship with your parents and siblings. These relationships, with their tensions and competitions, are deeply influential and birth order can often be matched to general personality features.

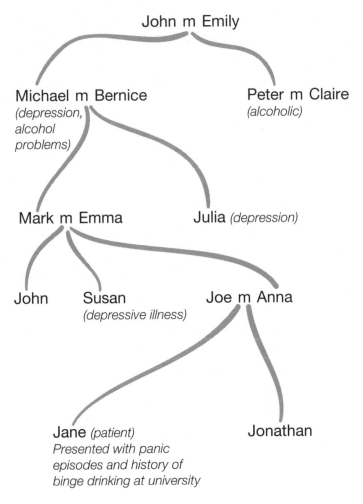

A typical geneagram

- **First-born.** You tend to be serious, conscientious, perfectionist and high achieving. As the eldest you often bore the weight of your parents' expectations. You were expected to behave better than the other children and had more responsibility placed on your shoulders. In adult life you can suffer from taking on too much, being overcautious and not thinking enough about yourself and your own needs.

- **Middle-born.** You tend to have a complex mix of sometimes contradictory characteristics – you are a mediator who dislikes conflict, and independent but fiercely loyal to your friends. You may be either easy-going or impatient. Middle children often feel under-appreciated or left out. In adult life you can be good at negotiating and compromise but may also lack assertiveness or feel bitter that you are not given enough attention.

STUCK IN THE MIDDLE

Judith, a woman in her sixties, was a middle-born child who told me she had 'grown up' at the age of six – when her youngest sister had come along. Both Judith's mother, who had been unwell, and her older sister were incapable of giving the baby all the care she needed, and it had fallen to Judith to do a lot of the nappy changing, feeding and soothing.

As a result, Judith felt stuck in the role of carer, unable to let rip and have fun as a child. She effectively lost part of her childhood by taking on an adult role far too soon. Middle children often find themselves becoming mediators within a family. Neither the favoured first-born nor the 'baby', they can get left out in the cold.

- **Last-born.** You tend to be charming, affectionate and outgoing but may also be manipulative, spoiled, impatient and wayward. As the baby of the family, last-born kids can also feel disempowered, with the consequence that in later life you may duck responsibility and expect to get away with more, and are more likely to go off the rails. Last-born kids, along with their middle-born siblings, may either be highly competitive with older siblings or avoid competition altogether by becoming opposites of older children; and middle-borns may also aim to occupy different roles from first-borns, for instance by becoming academic if the first-born is sporty. Each child in a family looks for ways to become unique and significant in their own right, in order to win parental approval and gain self-esteem – this is one of the roots of sibling rivalry.

- **Only children**. You are generally considered to have a mix of first and last-born characteristics. Like a first-born you bore the weight of parental expectation, but like a last-born you got all the attention and may have been spoiled. In adulthood you may become a perfectionist and find it hard to get on with contemporaries, and like a first-born you may need to lighten up and expect less of yourself.

- **Special cases**. These are broad generalisations, and some factors may change the picture altogether. For instance, siblings born more than five years apart may not occupy the same roles in relationship to one another, while gender influences can be significant. Children tend to identify more with siblings and parents of the same sex, while solitary boys in a group of girls may have their own issues, and vice versa.

Think about your place in the birth order and how it has influenced your personality and lifestyle. You may have carried these influences over into your adult life, or you may have fought hard to change or resist them. Either way, they have affected your choices, motivations and current lifestyle, so examining them can provide powerful insights.

Family atmosphere   Another major factor in childhood development is the atmosphere created by your parents in terms of their expectations and the ways in which they disciplined and rewarded you. Through their parenting style, parents provide children with a model of how to behave in order to win attention and affection. Most of us would like to think that we no longer live our lives in an attempt to please or gain attention from our parents, but as children we absorbed and internalised these models of behaviour. To an extent they will always be with us, guiding and motivating much of our behaviour.

Problem parenting styles   Even the best parents find it hard to always tread the fine line between being supportive but not smothering, firm but not repressive, motivating but not demanding. If these boundaries are regularly crossed, however, children can react by developing lifestyle characteristics that cause them problems in later life.

For instance, I have dealt with many patients who suffer from a pervasive sense of failure, stemming from demanding or overly critical parents. These are sometimes successful professionals from the tops of their fields complaining that they feel inadequate because they can't shake patterns that were laid down in childhood. Their parents always asked 'Why didn't you do better?' or found something to criticise. Not until they identify the sources of these feelings can they get past them, recognise their individual potential and achievements, and deal with physical or medical problems that relate to their emotional baggage. If you're a parent reading this you may recognise that you are the type to react badly if your superbright child gets a B (and is 'second best') when you know he's capable of an A! Once or twice I have found myself saying to one of my sons – who is normally top of the class – but why were you only third?!

Do you find that you are over-critical of yourself, or suffer from a different problem – over-competitiveness (driven by pure desire to win), neediness, fear of conflict, inability to say 'no', a constant desire to please, perhaps, or a fear of failure? Think about how your parents rewarded or disciplined you as a child.

Classroom and playground   When children venture into the wider world beyond the family environment, they transfer, or attempt to transfer, the social skills and strategies they have already learned. They also develop new skills and their lifestyles change accordingly. The classroom is where you first encountered adults and dealt with authority outside the family environment. The playground is where you extended your social world beyond your siblings, and it is here that you had to learn to negotiate the paths and pitfalls of society, making friends, joining groups and dealing with kids your own age. In Erikson's model of psychosocial development, the crisis of this stage is 'competence vs inferiority'. The challenge for the child is to develop belief in his or her own competence – perceived failure can lead to feelings of inferiority and low self-esteem. If you believe you can do it, you can build from that starting point.

Let's look at the playground first. The playground can be a great leveller, teaching spoiled or bossy children that life strategies that may work at home may cut no ice in the real world. Developing friendships, finding shared interests and building up a social network can boost a child's self-esteem and go some way towards compensating for an unsupportive family atmosphere. But the playground also has its hazards, particularly bullying, which can have traumatic and long-lasting effects. Low self-esteem, shyness and fear of self-expression are possible consequences. Emotional and psychological scars such as these inevitably affect a person's overall wellbeing. We compensate by trying to blend in, a basic survival instinct: trying to be like others. It takes courage to be an individual – for instance, a boy who likes to dance – as bullies will always see your Achilles' heel, be it that you're too clever, too tall, too small, too tidy or too talented.

The classroom can present other challenges and benefits. Sometimes one of my patients will mention a particular teacher, coach or other figure who stood out, illustrating that any adult, not just your parents, can act as a significant influence on your life. What is often more important, however, is how you were treated in class in general, because classroom experiences can have a great impact on your self-esteem and self-image. If you were encouraged at school and made to feel successful, you are more likely to be confident of your own abilities in later life. If, on the other hand, you were made to feel stupid or incapable, your self-esteem may have been badly damaged. Children who do not conform to the 'norm' in their peer group can also feel very isolated, or end up suppressing their true selves to fit in. This too can have a lasting negative effect.

Perhaps most important in both the classroom and family environment is the way mistakes were handled. Too many children learn not to risk trying new things because they are made to feel foolish or inadequate when they fail, and this can easily transfer into adult life. If your parents and teachers were supportive, you are more likely, as an adult, to be ready to risk change and innovation, and less likely to get stuck in a rut.

Puberty, adolescence, the teens

Teenage years have a bad rap as a time of confusion, assertion, anxiety and moodiness. Yet for many people, adolescence provides the best years of their lives. Undoubtedly, however, adolescence is a time of individuation – becoming an individual and defining one's individual identity. Many well-known aspects of adolescence relate to this process: joining a social group or 'tribe' (such as goth, jock, punk or raver); testing the boundaries of parental and school authority; exploring sexual identity. Some kids are always 'good' as teenagers – but will test life later on, maybe becoming promiscuous or experimenting with drugs in their twenties or thirties. You also get the classic 'perfect student' who then flunks his exams or gets sent down from university.

The most important thing is to have a family environment where defiance can be acted out safely.

Identity issues   Erikson described the conflict of this stage of life as being one of 'identity vs role confusion'. Role confusion is better known as 'identity crisis' – a state where you're not sure who you are, where you belong or what you want to do. This conflict is a good example of one that often recurs in later life, particularly in this day and age when people take a lot longer to 'settle down' – to pick a career, start a family and stick with them. An increasing number of people don't know what they want to do or where they want to go with their lives, and many others find that they've made these decisions too early, and now feel 'trapped' by them or afraid to change course. A typical example is John, who'd found himself stuck in a career in engineering, just because that was what his family expected of him. He'd always actually wanted to be a chef – but this course was frowned upon by his parents.

Have you resolved this conflict in your life? Are you confident and secure in your identity? I find that a lot of my patients have problems that ultimately stem from challenges to their identity – they thought they knew what they wanted and where they were going, but for one reason or another have come to reassess their priorities. The resulting psychological uncertainty can manifest itself as a general malaise, a chronic sense of 'not feeling 100 per cent'.

Fitting in and standing out   One of the positive aspects of adolescence is developing a network of social support outside your family. By doing this you affirm both your individuality and your self-worth – in other words, you feel good about yourself. Plus, of course, you have fun with your friends (of both sexes). Not fitting in or being accepted, however, is one of a teenager's greatest sources of anxiety. A major factor in determining whether you fit in or stand out is a biological one – the onset of puberty.

Boys and girls who enter puberty significantly earlier or later than their peers can experience problems. Studies show that early maturing boys and girls initially develop more positive views of themselves and become more popular with their peers, but may be more likely to end up with behavioural or emotional difficulties. Late developers may tend to have a more negative view of themselves, and although their self-esteem generally catches up, particularly late developers may be left with long-term feelings of inferiority. Think about the timing of your puberty – did it cause problems for you?

Rebellion   As a child, your identity is defined in large part by membership of a family group (one reason why children from dysfunctional or fragmented families are likely to have so many problems). As an adolescent, a key part of the process of developing your individual identity is defining it in opposition to your family – specifically your parents, and by extension other authority figures such as teachers. But in reacting automatically against your parents and their values and aspirations, you might not end up being true to yourself.

For instance, if you left school early because you couldn't wait to get a job and move out, you might have deprived yourself of further education that you actually wanted. Or perhaps you took up smoking or drinking just because they told you not to, only to find out later that, of course, they were right. How would you describe your relationship with your parents? Were they permissive or strict? Research indicates that the most successful parenting style is somewhere in between – authoritative but not authoritarian. Where were your parents on this scale? Could their parenting style have affected your present-day habits or lifestyle? Did you feel loved, essentially 'secure'?

BAND AID

Michael was a successful executive in his mid-thirties who had come to see me not because of any specific illness, but simply because he hadn't felt 'well' for some time and was fed up with this constant sense of malaise. As we went through his Potted Life History, it was his adolescent years that came to the fore – this was clearly the part of his life he recalled with

---

greatest affection. He had been a gifted musician and songwriter, and in his late teenage years he and a group of friends had had a band and performed around the city with some success, despite the disapproval of his parents. Eventually pressures had led the band to break up and, encouraged by his parents, Michael had focused more and more on his career, achieving rapid promotion and getting caught up in work.

We agreed that this early life choice had resulted in him suppressing an important facet of his personality – his creativity. For many years he had failed to recognise the harm this suppression was doing, but now it was taking the shine off other aspects of his life. He decided to try and rekindle some of his creative spark by hiring a room every Friday night and getting some friends together for rehearsal. We also worked on his diet and lifestyle, taking the whole of his health triangle into account. Several months later he was feeling better again, and he and his band were even talking about putting together an album.

Coping with divorce A high proportion of my patients come from families that have broken up for various reasons, a background that often gives them extra issues to deal with. In the case of divorce, the issues may depend on when their parents' divorce happened and how it was handled. Studies show that if parents are arguing and fighting, children can often end up unhappier and more disturbed if they do not separate. If your parents split up when you were between around 8 and 16, however, you are likely to have been hit particularly hard. Contact with one of your parents may have been severely curtailed and this could leave you with unresolved anger and anxiety for many years, feelings that can affect your choice of partners and success at relationships in your adult life.

When taking a life history from a patient whose parents were divorced, I look for information on their age at the time of the split, the resulting parenting arrangements, the atmosphere of subsequent relations between the parents, and the presence of step-parents or step-siblings. Simply talking about these facts can open avenues for more revealing discussions, uncovering feelings or issues that may bear on their medical problems.

A lot of patients say to me: 'Everything was going fine until . . . ' And often that 'until' turns out to be their parents' divorce, which may have resulted in them seeing less of one parent, very often their father. Children crave what I call 'ordinary time' with both parents – the everyday stuff, not just so-called 'quality time' outings packed into one weekend. We cannot create a world without divorce and separation, but we can be aware of the issues as they may have affected us in the past, or as they may affect both the adults and children involved in the present.

CHAPTER 16

Growing up

The main challenge of young adulthood is to reconcile the need for intimacy and companionship, which requires commitment and compromise, with the enjoyment of being independent. As we discussed above, the 'identity vs role confusion' conflict of adolescence can also be a defining feature of adulthood. Assuming that you have already lived a good number of years, you may have been wrestling with these issues for some time, but perhaps not consciously – after all, most people simply get on with their lives without too much introspection. Now, however, I'd like you to engage in a bit of introspection, and think about some of the choices you've made.

Turning points

What was the route that led to where and who you are today? Your personality and lifestyle, your career, home and relationships are all the result of a unique series of choices, actions and indeed omissions. These important and formative moments could be called turning points, because if you'd made different choices your life could have been set on a different route. I look for these turning points in my patients' life histories because they may and often do reveal hidden regrets and unfulfilled desires, which act as emotional anchors weighing the person down with consequences for their mental and physical health.

Think about the turning points in your own life (often 'the best thing I ever did!'). What would have happened if you'd followed an alternative route? Do you have emotional anchors, unresolved issues or unfulfilled dreams? Did you take the safer bet? All this could be linked to your present-day state of health and levels of wellbeing.

Career choice and development

Look back over your career to date and think about how you arrived at where you are now. Over the years your job will have had a powerful influence over a range of psychological and physical issues such as self-esteem, mood, structural health and biochemical health.

A lucky few people have been able to do a job that perfectly combines security with creative and fulfilling work. Most of the rest of us have had to make some degree of compromise, which isn't the end of the world. If, however, you found yourself stuck in a rut or enduring poor conditions for long periods, your psychological and physical health may have suffered. Feeling that you are locked into a negative cycle can be depressing and debilitating. It saps your reserves of mental and therefore vital energy, undermines confidence, and, as we discussed above, may translate into chronic illness. If you were unhappy with your job then it may well have also made you unhealthy.

LISTEN TO YOUR INNER LONGINGS

Katherine was in her early forties when she came to see me. She was a natural academic, at her happiest when researching in obscure European libraries – but this purely academic life didn't make her a decent living, and, keen not to live like an eternal student, she took a job as a translator. When she came to see me she was comfortably off, but realised her career choice had hugely compromised her natural tendency. For a year or so she felt anxious, introspective, hypochondriachal, and rather lonely. Finally realising she had to satisfy her craving for obscure Latin tomes, she involved herself in a research project and now has contact with like minds. This was still something of a compromise, but more satisfying for Katherine. She is happier at work now, and, as a result, her introspection and health anxieties have resolved.

Think also about the working environment you've experienced in your life. Was it a positive one, with good air and light, good ergonomics and supportive relationships with colleagues? Environments like this can compensate for a less than satisfactory job, while ones without these positive features simply add a structural and biochemical burden to your psychological one.

Making the wrong choice   We are all multi-faceted individuals, with many different talents and abilities. The process of choosing and pursuing a career often involves polishing one facet of yourself – the one the world usually sees – and neglecting others, such as your creative abilities. If you have neglected some facets of your personality, perhaps through making a career choice that you were never truly comfortable with, your health could suffer.

The mating game

Finding a partner is important to most people's long-term happiness, but that doesn't mean it's easy. Rewarding and stable relationships help to boost your reserves of self-esteem and positive energy, but your romantic history will almost inevitably contain disappointments and heartache. How you dealt with these may have affected how you view relationships and life in the present day.

A history of hurtful rejections, for instance, may have battered your self-esteem and left you with a negative self-image. Damaging or dysfunctional relationships take a psychological toll, as do bad break-ups. Many psychologists liken getting over a significant relationship to coping with bereavement. You have to go through the same stages of grief and acceptance, and maybe anger, if you are to have peace of mind. Failing to progress through these stages can make it hard for you move on, providing another potential source of emotional baggage.

Parenthood

The issue of having children features quite heavily in the life histories of many of my patients, although often they are more conspicuous by their absence. The crisis of mature adulthood is a conflict between your comfortable, settled life and the need to express yourself, be creative and bring new things into the world, even though this may upset your carefully ordered life, just when you had everything set up the way you want it. The way most people try to resolve this conflict is by having children.

Reward and responsibility The positive aspects of parenting bring joy, reciprocated love and fulfilment, charging up your emotional batteries and giving you strong family and social roots. The negative aspects include financial and emotional stress, self-compromise and strain on your relationship with your partner. If you've had children, think about how it affected issues as diverse as your sleeping patterns, your love life and your ability to pursue your own dreams and goals.

Consider also the health issues that surrounded the process. How did you feel about your or your partner's pregnancy, labour, breastfeeding and sleepless nights; about your body or your partner's body? Apart from their clinical aspects, these issues often throw up important emotional and psychological issues.

Termination issues Terminated pregnancies are a common feature of modern life, and in general society seems not to make too much fuss over them. Perhaps surprisingly, then, I have found that unresolved issues surrounding terminations can be a major problem for many of my patients (both men and women).

Women who had a termination years ago, who may have felt huge relief at the time, can be almost reduced to tears when they reach this part of their life history. It turns out they've been carrying a lot of suppressed emotion for all that time – unconscious sadness and suppressed anxiety about future fertility. Some of my male patients who may have easily accepted a termination at the time have also reassessed their feelings about it as years have gone by. Not surprisingly, such reassessments and regrets are strongest in those who find themselves beyond child-rearing age, or in a childless relationship (see 'The biological clock', page 233).

Issues like these can become sources of subconscious unease, making you chronically unhappy or discontented without knowing why – and possibly contributing to chronic physical malaise. In order to deal with these problems, you need to bring them out into the open by thinking and talking about them in a safe and supportive environment.

Mature adult, middle age and retirement

There's not much of a dividing line between young adulthood and middle years, particularly today when working lives are longer and 40 or even 50 is the 'new 30'. Nonetheless, there are three areas of concern that stand out for those old enough to look back on their middle years – retirement, the 'empty nest' syndrome and, for women, menopause.

Retirement

Reaching the end of your working life is a major life event. No matter how well prepared you are, retirement has the potential to reawaken old crises, and the way in which people cope with them says a lot about their reserves of mental and vital energy.

The most obvious effect of retirement is that it threatens to rekindle the perennial problem of identity. If you have defined yourself in large part through your career, who do you become when that career is over? If you've thrown everything into your job and devoted little time to outside interests you may not be left with much. The same issues apply to homemakers or full-time parents experiencing empty nest syndrome (see below).

Revisiting adolescent-style identity crises can be very disorienting for grown men and women who thought they were past all that, and having to renegotiate an identity later in life is a real challenge – especially if their relationship is also being reviewed. Depending on how well people manage it, they could be contemplating security and peace of mind in older age, or struggling with continued role confusion, with obvious consequences for their peace of mind. If you are a retiree, ask yourself how you felt on your retirement. Were you well prepared for it? Did it feel different to the way you expected it to be? Did you feel you had lost status? Did it change the way you saw and/or described yourself?

Did it change how you were viewed by your partner and friends? Did you feel 'put out to grass'?

RETIREMENT AND RELATIONSHIPS

Margaret, a very 'Home Counties' lady, told me how much she disliked her husband's attitude and outlook since his retirement. Outgoing and interesting while still a senior manager in a multinational company, he had become, once retired, completely obsessed with the Internet. She had also left her career to enjoy their early retirement together – and ended up deeply frustrated. The situation was deteriorating and she told me that far from growing together in retirement, they had grown apart. So she had left their comfortable home and moved away to study. Other couples manage to make the move to retirement together, but extra effort is needed to address the profound issues that will certainly arise.

As for family, we worry about children when they are little, when they are growing up, and when they leave home. That 'empty nest' feeling can hit parents very hard indeed. One patient of mine is a lovely lady who is a devoted wife and superb mother of very successful children. When the children had all left home, her husband was very supportive, but she found it extremely difficult coping with an empty house. She found herself crying at the supermarket, just longing for her daughter to return home in the holidays. Letting go isn't easy.

My own children want to develop specialist music and acting careers that will mean both of them sometimes living a long way from our family home, and travelling a great deal. They are hugely loved and confident in this and I know it's my role to always be there for them and support them through the ups and downs. Living together for ever was never an option and it shouldn't be, but I've every sympathy with the 'empty nest' feeling. We have to let our children go, and try not to worry ourselves to distraction about them.

With advancing years, physical and sexual problems can also come to the fore. One couple came to see me a few months after the husband had retired from a very successful City directorship. When he was working, he'd had little time for much else, and their sex life had become non-existent. This they had blamed on their lifestyle, and his work. But these 'causes' were actually excuses; with plenty of time on their hands, they found they were unable to rekindle the flames, because they had swept the real reasons for the demise of their physical relationship under the carpet. We therefore sat down and discussed all the issues, to determine how to get things going once more.

Another recently retired man came to see me as he was worried about his heart. It turned out that he'd been concerned about the possibility of suffering a coronary for some years, but hadn't wanted this to affect his work or promotion prospects. He had been particularly concerned not to jeopardise his health insurance prospects – which he would have to take out when the cover that came with his job ceased. So many men suffer collapses in health soon after retirement, as if they cannot cope with no longer being working people. Although some of this may be due to a sudden decline in their feelings of status and general usefulness, the neglect of their health while working is the more significant reason. Stopping work also removes men from the social environment in which they spend most of their time, and social contacts which are clearly defined. Men are not as socially adept as women and can become isolated more easily. Loneliness can lead to depression, and further problems such as eating badly or drinking too much.

Having a comprehensive health check in advance of retirement is a very important preparatory move – more important even than reading up on the relative merits of annuities, and booking the world cruise. You really don't want to end up being flown back from Barbados following a heart attack . . .

Productivity

Doing a job, no matter what, makes you feel productive – you're doing a day's work and being paid for it. Relaxing and enjoying your leisure are obviously important features of retirement, but feeling unproductive can be demoralising, even if you're not consciously aware of it. Many retirees find alternative avenues for their productivity. Gardening, working for a charity, looking after grandchildren – these are all examples of attempts to rechannel the urge to be productive or nurturing. Finding an outlet for your productivity and creativity is vital for achieving mental equilibrium.

Think about how you have expressed your need for generativity since retirement.

The empty nest

When the kids grow up, become independent and move out, you may be left with an empty house and many of the same issues that are posed by retirement. Parents are thrown back on their own resources and, as we discussed above, once again find themselves defining new identities. If your children have moved out, do you feel liberated or lonely? Has it made you reassess your priorities?

Another common issue for retirees is anxiety over the changing roles of both partners in the home, a situation that can be complicated by empty nest issues. If you are the homemaker, how did you accommodate a partner who was suddenly around all the time? If you had previously been the breadwinner, did you feel out of place and underfoot? Again, these are issues of identity and role confusion.

The menopause

Just as women have different physical experiences of menopause, so they react differently in psychological terms. For some women it can be a time of sadness, as they mourn their lost fertility, or a time of identity confusion, as they feel their femininity threatened. Other women feel liberated, or a mixture of these things. Either way, the menopause marks a distinct and biologically underlined transition, and major transitions inevitably change and upset your dynamic equilibrium. After a period of flux it should settle down into a new but equally stable equilibrium.

Men share many of the same feelings of regret and identity confusion. Because of many men's reluctance to discuss their feelings and the general lack of awareness about emotions men experience as they get older, many men may feel isolated.

How well and positively you move into your more mature years depends on a number of factors, including your self-esteem, the stability of your identity and the support of friends and relations. One of the biggest factors affecting how a woman moves through menopause is whether she is childless or child free, and if so, how she feels about that. For some childless women, with or without partners, impending menopause comes as a wake-up call, but sadly, often too late. This can be very distressing, with severe consequences for both psychological and physical health. For others, who are secure in their choice to remain childless or who have accepted that they will not have children, menopause is not such a big deal. If you were childless at menopause, which category did you fall into? How did you cope?

MENOPAUSE: RELIEF OR REGRET?

Sooner or later during a woman's forties, she will approach the menopause, leading up to the time that the monthly release of an egg from the ovaries and monthly periods cease. The age at which a woman reaches menopause may reflect that of her mother, so it is useful to find out if your mother had a particularly early or late menopause. Some women will welcome the menopause, especially if they have had particularly heavy or painful periods. Others will think nothing of it and be happy with their lot, moving with ease into the period-free stage of their lives.

Menopause is nevertheless a time of physical change and emotional issues. There are the short-term health issues that need to be discussed: hot flushes, poor sleep, changes in libido and vaginal dryness; and the long-term issues like planning for a healthy future free of osteoporosis and other conditions that are more common after the menopause.

One woman I know well, an artist, felt it was a voyage of discovery – a new equilibrium and a powerful feeling that she had arrived safely to the next stage of womanhood. She doesn't have children and is very comfortable with this, explaining that she feels her creativity is expressed through her art.

Another felt bereaved over the loss of her fertility. She had four teenage children and a happy life, had never considered having a baby in her forties and knew how blessed she was to have children and the prospect of grandchildren. But the knowledge that she would never hold her own baby again saddened her.

Of course, for others who have wanted children and for whom it just hasn't happened, menopause can be a very difficult time. Sometimes it is

---

because the man, or the woman, or both, suffer from subfertility. Sometimes a relationship has just never arrived at the right point for both to want to have children.

One woman in her early forties at last met the man of her dreams, but sadly her menopause was early – as her mother's had been before her – and she was not able to conceive. However, neither partner had based their hopes for a successful marriage on children, and I think they will be happy loving each other for their own sakes.

Old age

The crisis that older people have to resolve is often an existential one. Young people can be uncertain of their identities, but totally unaware of their mortality; death is something that happens to others. In old age this is reversed: we come to understand ourselves but may despair of the future. It can become a stand-off between finding wisdom and tranquillity through acceptance of your life, and giving in to fears or negative thoughts of your own mortality.

Intimations of mortality

The possibilities of illness and death become more likely prospects in older age, and this can be, naturally, quite frightening. Anxiety over ill health can profoundly affect your peace of mind. Distress can lead to apathy and despair, which in turn can lead to low energy levels and a depressed immune system – fear of illness may become a self-fulfilling prophecy.

In fact, I find that abrupt and distressing awareness of mortality is something that can strike at any life stage. Among my patients it typically affects adults in their middle years experiencing serious illness or surgery, possibly for the first time, or waiting for the results of serious health tests – such as breast lump biopsies. Sometimes older people are much better equipped to deal with these anxieties, thanks to their store of experience and knowledge, and their ability to face serious issues with equanimity. How do you feel about these weighty issues?

Ageing gracefully

The infirmity of extreme old age also marks a kind of return to the physical status of infancy. In psychosocial terms, we could say that extreme old age revives the crisis of childhood – the desire to be independent vs fear and embarrassment over dependency. My aim is to make this less of a problem. I want older people to enjoy good health for longer. By living a healthy active life, risks of infirmity and dependence are reduced. Scourges like osteoporosis, falls and fractures, embarrassing incontinence, heart disease and cancers are less likely to affect those who have actively worked to prevent them.

The improving health of the elderly has, in fact, led to a reassessment of our notions about old age, and a realisation that many of the problems we traditionally associate with this time of life are social rather than biological. Older people who remain active and engaged, interact with others and are allowed a role in the community instead of being passed over enjoy a better quality of life and retain their intellectual and physical abilities for longer.

If you are past the age of 70, the challenge for you is to maintain the reserves of vital energy that will keep you going, through engaging in intellectual, physical and social pursuits. If you are below this age, the challenge is to build up your reserves so that they will serve you well in later life.

Where are you now?

If you've read through the previous section, and used it as a jumping-off point for thinking about your own history, then hopefully you've started to think about how you got to where you are today. But I don't believe that we are entirely defined by our pasts. Although past history is important and often underappreciated as an influence on our habits, motivations and behaviour, each of us is a free-willed individual with the capacity to make choices and determine our own actions in the present day, and we are fully responsible for those choices and actions. Ultimately, this means that you are directly and immediately responsible for your present and future peace of mind. This is why, as well as reviewing your past, it's also important to look at your life in the present.

CHAPTER 17

Your emotional lifestyle

We've already discussed some aspects of lifestyle in previous chapters – for instance, diet, activity levels and alcohol consumption. Here I'd like to look at the wider issues of mental equilibrium, and the effect on your whole health triangle. Two factors, stress and self-fulfilment, have a major influence on your physical and mental wellbeing. Your career, your life outside your career, and the balance between the two, are intimately linked to both these factors.

Stress

When you think of stress, the thought may conjure up traffic jams, commuter hassle, tight deadlines, irritating neighbours and the like. Well, yes, these are all sources of stress, but over the last few decades the term 'stress' has taken on a wider meaning in the world of health psychology. In its broader sense, it refers to anything that drains your emotional reserves and/or threatens your mental equilibrium. As you can imagine, this is a very broad definition – it includes everything from having your home repossessed or losing a loved one, to living on a noisy street or coping with a bad relationship.

Psychologists and doctors alike have come to realise that stress is one of the single most important factors determining your mental and physical health, possibly playing a role in deciding who may be more likely to get diseases like cancer or atherosclerosis.

But there are many varieties of stress, and not all of them are negative. Many stressful activities can be enjoyable – watching a horror movie or clinching a business deal, for instance – and some people thrive on stress. Patients of mine in the banking sector, for instance, commonly describe their jobs as both extremely stressful and very enjoyable. They love it! In purely physiological terms, we may need at least some stress to keep our system in prime condition, and, in psychological terms, it is through experiencing stress and coping with it that we grow and mature.

Your response to stress

The first studies on the link between stress and illness uncovered confusing results. In some people there was a direct correlation between stress and ill health, while in others the picture was less clear. Since then, researchers have come to appreciate that the individual's response to stress, rather than the stress itself, is the important factor (obvious, really, although not to sufferers).

How do you respond to stress? The answer could provide a useful insight into your ability to achieve peace of mind and associated good health. Response to stress depends on a number of personality features:

- **Temperament.** During the 1970s it was widely believed that Type A personalities – irritable, impatient high achievers – responded badly to stress, but research showed that this was not universally true. Instead it seems that one trait in particular makes you react badly to stress: hostility. People who are chronically hostile – that is, more likely to think the worst of people, have arguments, get resentful or be unpleasant – are more likely to get ill because of stress. People with depression also respond badly to stress.

- **Repression.** Do you try to repress anxiety, fear and other negative emotions, or are you willing to think and talk about them, looking for practical approaches and solutions? It's true that dwelling on things in isolation that you can't do anything about isn't helpful, and can in fact increase your stress levels. In general, however, people who try to avoid facing stressful thoughts or emotions – and so do not get on with understanding them and seeking solutions – usually fare worse than more expressive people.

- **Optimism and pessimism.** When people talk or think about the causes of stress they can adopt one of two 'explanatory styles' – optimistic or pessimistic. For instance, failure is a source of stress, but an optimistic person will respond better to failure because they may blame it on circumstances rather than themselves, and be positive about the future – the 'it won't happen next time' approach. Pessimistic people tend to have lower self-esteem and more illness – in other words, they have lower reserves of emotional energy.

- **Sense of control.** Another factor is how much of a sense of control you have over a source of stress. Feeling that you have no control can make you respond much worse to stress. For instance, most people have to cope with some level of office politics. If it's a colleague that's causing you trouble you might not feel too bad – after all, you can always challenge them if you need to. If it's your boss, on the other hand, you might feel there's nothing you can do, and you'll be more likely to perceive your office environment as hostile and negative, and to be stressed by it – rather than energised.

Coping styles   Supposing that you are a pessimistic person, or prone to react with hostility – does this mean you're doomed to be stressed out for the rest of your life? Is a personality transplant necessary if you want to avoid the damaging effects of stress? No! Just because you don't respond well to stress, doesn't mean you can't learn to cope with it. In fact almost all of us already use a variety of 'coping styles' to mitigate the effects of stress, though with varying degrees of success. We'll be looking at the different coping styles and talking about how you can acquire them in Chapter 18.

A sense of balance

I've talked enough about the importance of the health triangle and the various components of your life which contribute to its equilibrium. One of these components, your lifestyle, is also made up of various ingredients –

your career, your home and social life, your hobbies and pastimes, and so on – which need to be harmoniously balanced if your life is to be happy and healthy.

Success in your chosen career is a major source of fulfilment. At the most basic level, it is good for your self-esteem to provide for yourself and do well at something, and hopefully your work gives you all this and more. Devoting time and energy to your career is therefore an important step in achieving a harmonious lifestyle balance. Increasingly, however, people are expected to work longer and longer hours, throwing their lifestyles out of balance.

OVERWORKED AND UNDER-RELAXED

People in the UK have the shortest holidays and the longest working hours in Europe. However Australians, New Zealanders and North Americans all work even longer hours than their British counterparts – and with similar or fewer holidays. With the majority wishing they could have a better work/life balance, but fearing their career and hard-earned status would suffer if they pushed for fewer hours, it's a real concern.

This is a common pattern among my patients – driven, career-oriented men and women who cannot understand why they feel subliminally discontented despite the success they have achieved by 'normal' standards. One problem here is obviously the notion of 'normal' standards of success, which usually translate as material success – promotion, perks, salary. These norms represent a pretty, one-sided view of life's priorities but one that has unfortunately taken a firm hold on our society, contributing to the pressure to spend more and work harder. Perhaps our standards of success should be more individualised – they should certainly be more balanced. What's your own definition of 'success'? Could it be improved upon? Are you fulfilled and enjoying life?

Very often the career men and women I see who are discontented do not have well-balanced lifestyles. They concentrate too much on work and assume the rest of their life will take care of itself. Some of them may have made a conscious choice not to spend time looking for relationships or developing other parts of themselves; others may simply not have time. But neglecting the non-career parts of your life is a false economy, at least in psychological terms. Someone whose lifestyle reflects a balance between their different needs and responsibilities will be more self-fulfilled and therefore likely to be ultimately more effective in all aspects of their life – including work. Indeed, employers may seek people who are effective at work *and* 'have a life'!

How many hours a week do you work? How often do you work through lunch/into the evening/at weekends? Are you planning to slow down 'in the future' or concentrate on your career for the next 10/20/30 years until you're comfortably off and then think about other things? Do you find yourself squeezing hobbies, sport or other pastimes into rigidly defined slots in your calendar, or even having to skip them altogether? In Chapters 19 and 20 we'll talk about how you can use your limited time to best effect, and discuss putting things in perspective, reassessing priorities and developing other facets of your life.

Beyond the grind

Even workaholics know that there should be more to life than the daily grind. I've already mentioned some obvious balancers, like sport, hobbies or relationships, and you can probably think of loads of things that you could do for your own enjoyment or education. But like the materialistic values we talked about above, these are elements of life that involve looking inwards – focusing on the individual, and concerned only with what is personal.

I believe that by only 'looking in' we lose sight of many other aspects of life, which can be equally important to achieving a balanced lifestyle. Paradoxically, we also need to 'look outwards' to achieve self-fulfilment. That can mean many different things – interacting more with your community, volunteering for a charity, getting involved at your kids' school or passing on your skills and experience through some teaching of your own. The World Health Organization's definition of health as 'a state of complete physical, mental and *social* wellbeing' recognises this outward-looking dimension as important to health, particularly as it avoids one of the fundamental psychological risks of adult life – stagnation.

Take a moment to review your lifestyle with respect to this 'in-out' dimension. How much of your life involves looking out? Are you involved in your local community or in a charitable or teaching organisation? In the work I do with people planning retirement I find that among senior managers, many of their retirement plans involve just this sort of outward-looking activity. But do you have to wait until retirement to shift your focus slightly? By putting it off you could effectively post-date part of your self-fulfilment.

LOOKING OUT – FOR SELF AND OTHERS

Many of my patients have benefited from altruism.

Simon, a success in banking, had already made loads of money by his late twenties. He had his Porsche, waterside home, and all the other trappings he needed, but wanted to use his skills to help other people as well. After a long chat with me, he contacted a local school for disabled children and is now on their board of governors, advising on financial issues. He finds this hugely satisfying, and this unpaid work for the school has become an important part of his life.

Alison, a company secretary, is also financially secure and in a good job. And, for some years now, she has worked on a voluntary basis for a few hours every week, helping to feed elderly ladies. This satisfies her caring nature and fulfils a real need.

Responsibilities

As well as making sure you have some freedom from responsibility – time to play – it's also important to make sure you have enough responsibility in your life. Too little can leave you feeling rootless or vulnerable, too much can make you feel stifled or overburdened. Responsibilities can disturb your mental equilibrium through their absence as well as their presence, and many of my younger patients feel anxious because they are not keeping pace with the 'social clock' – the timetable of major life events that society has traditionally decreed as 'usual' or 'standard'. For instance, you may feel that you are lagging behind the social clock if you're approaching 30 and haven't got a house or settled on a career because you're still studying, travelling or simply haven't found a vocation. Alternatively, you might feel that you've got ahead of the social clock if you're staying in to change nappies while your mates are out clubbing.

Do you feel the pressure of the social clock? Does being 'out of sync' bother you? Remember that the anxieties caused by the social clock stem mainly from our perceptions and our need to conform. There is no definitive or standard social clock. You have to define your own timetable – unless it is individually tailored, you could end up 'out of sync' with yourself.

The biological clock

The one major exception to this rule is the issue of fertility. While the social clock is gradually changing and more people leave having children until later, a woman's fertility follows its own biological clock, and no amount of individual tailoring can change that. One result is the declining birth rate in this country, which has dropped from 2.4 children per couple to 1.8 over the last decade or so. The human face of this demographic change is an increasing number of childless late thirty- and early fortysomethings.

Many of my patients are 'child-free' women, beyond child-bearing age. Some have no regrets and feel fulfilled and productive. Others, however, are not so happy. Some of them took a conscious decision not to have kids, and now regret it bitterly. Others were too busy getting on with the rest of their lives and took it for granted that there would be time 'later'. Sadly, some are now left reassessing their priorities, but too late. Some of my older male patients are in a similar situation – they went along with their partners' decision not to have kids, but now regret it.

Disappointment on this scale can carry a severe psychological penalty. I've already mentioned the psychological clash between the need to be creative and stagnation in adult life, and the crisis that occurs when creativity, particularly through reproducing children, imposes itself. My childless patients who are contented and self-fulfilled have generally found other ways to resolve this crisis, pursuing other outlets for their creativity. But for many men and women there is no substitute for children.

Have you given serious thought to the realities of your biological clock?

Do you know the facts about female fertility? Do you reassure yourself that, if it came to it, you would rely on assisted conception techniques such as IVF treatment or frozen eggs, when the truth is that these techniques only work for a small minority? This may all sound a bit alarmist, but I see so many women who are 38 or so and still tell me, 'I'm not ready for a baby just yet – maybe in a couple of years.' In a couple of years, it may no longer be as straightforward.

When Diana first came to me, in her late thirties, she was so caught up in her business career that the issue of when to have children still seemed years off. One day a few years later, she came to me saying that the urge to reproduce had finally clicked in, and that she and her partner were now ready. She was concerned that her periods were very irregular, however, and blood tests revealed that she was clearly menopausal. The moment had passed and it was now too late. Assisted conception techniques and paying attention to lifestyle may result in a successful pregnancy, but the chances are far lower than for a younger woman.

If you know for sure that you want kids and you are in your thirties, you need to be careful about the assumptions you make about your fertility. Don't view it too casually, and above all, don't procrastinate. Be aware, too, that there's never a 'perfect time' to have children. If you want them, you will find ways of accommodating this ultimate responsibility in your life.

Relationships

We've already discussed the issue of past relationships and their emotional legacy. In this section I'd like you to take a look at your current relationships – not just your romantic ones, but also the ones you have with your friends and family. The quality of your relationships is crucial to your mental wellbeing.

Positive relationships boost your emotional wellbeing by enhancing your self-esteem and helping you to cope with stress. Negative ones have the opposite effect, yet many people find themselves stuck in a damaging relationship, or constantly moving from one to the other. Why do some people seem to be bad at picking partners or maintaining quality relationships? You may find yourself in a pattern of damaging relationships – where does it come from? Could it have anything to do with your family relationships, or are there other factors?

Hayley told me how her childhood had been unhappy since her parents had separated when she was eight. She felt a need to nurture in her relationships, and ended up with three consecutive boyfriends who took her for granted – letting her do all their cooking and shopping, and not sharing the financial costs. Worse still, a couple of them became verbally and physically abusive towards her.

We've seen how important childhood, and family, are to development. Persistent patterns of behaviour in your adult life often result from templates in your subconscious – prototypes of how to behave that were laid down at times in your life when you were particularly impressionable, usually childhood. And when it comes to relationships, for most people the basis for these templates is their parents' relationship.

For example, if your parents had a warm, affectionate relationship with lots of hugs and kisses, you might have picked up on this as a template for the future. If they had a stormy, passionate relationship with lots of fights, or bitter 'point scoring', you might find yourself repeating this pattern. Think about how your parents interacted and then think about your own relationships. Can you see similarities?

You are not preordained to copy your parents directly. Their example might prompt you to avoid aspects of your parents' relationship that you particularly disliked, or seek out qualities you felt were missing, in your own relationships. For instance, you might look for a quiet, stable partnership because you are subconsciously reacting against the stormy relationship you had to cope with as a child.

Somewhat scarily, the template theory also means that for most people the template for your ideal partner – the subconscious image against which potential partners are checked and rated – comes from your parent! So if you find yourself attracted to cold, distant women, or clinging, dependent men, think about your mother or father, respectively. Were they like this, or perhaps the opposite?

Sex

When Freud first started talking about the subconscious and its drives, he focused on sex as the dominant factor. Roughly a hundred years later, sex, though no longer as prominent in psychological theory, still dominates much of our thinking. Issues of self-esteem and gender identity are closely tied to sexuality, so sexual problems can profoundly affect mental wellbeing far beyond the bedroom.

As a doctor, I deal with a lot of sexual problems that are biological in origin but psychological in consequence. Failure to sustain an erection, for instance, may be linked to medication taken for high blood pressure, but its consequences can include relationship anxieties, fears about sexuality and doubts about masculinity. Performance anxiety can exacerbate low libido and depression. And the process can work in reverse. I've had cases where repression of a sexual problem has given rise to physical symptoms – what psychiatrists call a conversion symptom.

One man in his fifties was referred to me after extensive investigation of intractable headaches. After several consultations, his emotional history revealed he'd been cross-dressing in his wife's clothes for years – and had always felt guilty. Sensitive counselling helped him regain peace of mind and a feeling of 'comfortableness' within himself . . . and his symptoms were gradually resolved.

A look at your sex life   Because sex is so important in our lives, during an initial consultation I ask patients whether they have any concerns about their sex lives. Equally, when you are reviewing your life in this chapter you should give some thought to sex. Some issues may have come up during your Potted Life History – for instance, how you first learned about sex, whether you ever had doubts about your sexual orientation and when you lost your virginity. Think about how any issues may have affected your present-day sex life and attitudes towards sex.

How would you rate your sex life? What makes it good, bad or indifferent, and what are you comparing it to? In fact, it's very hard to rate your sex life by any objective scale, because who is to say what's normal? You have to make the judgement for yourself, according to your perception, experience and expectations, and it's these that sometimes cause trouble.

Your expectations date back to your earliest education about sex and, later, to your first experiences, but they may not be serving you well. Our culture typically encourages unrealistic expectations – for instance, that both partners should reach orgasm every time they have sex, or that penetrative intercourse is the only 'real' form of sex. Do you need to review your expectations?

Your perceptions about your sex life may not match up with your partner's, and this can be another source of problems. Any sex therapist will tell you that good communication is the key to successful sex, and to successful resolution of sexual problems. How good is your communication with your partner? Are you really expressing yourself physically, do you feel comfortable with and understand your partner's desires, and are you meeting your needs?

This last question is very important. Some people are too shy to discuss this and may then find more satisfaction in 'solo' sex than with their partner – a rather isolating state of affairs. Sometimes a woman will tell me that sometimes she just wants to be close to and to feel loved by her partner, but he always embarks on adventurous, vigorous sex sessions which she doesn't always enjoy – and of course, vice versa.

Your social network

No man is an island, as the poet John Donne said – we are all part of a support base. Your social network, comprised of your friends and family, is also a safety net. Very few people are true loners. But this is another area where so many people get their priorities out of order. I regularly see patients who are successful yet lonely people, whether or not they can consciously admit it. An intense focus on material priorities has led them to neglect other areas of their lives, unbalancing their lifestyle and therefore their psychological equilibrium. Take a moment to reassess the role that your social network plays in your life. How would it affect you if you lost it?

Some of my younger patients seem to be caught in a pattern of serial monogamy, where they have a serious relationship which ultimately fails maybe because of a fear of commitment by one or both sides. (And contrary to what many people imagine, commitment-phobia is not exclusive to men. Women can also seem more focused on themselves than on their relationships.) Being in an uncommited long-term relationship can drain your emotional reserves, because however enjoyable it is, there will always be a lurking insecurity at the back of your mind. Loyalty and trust in your partner's loyalty are crucial to the health of a relationship and its influence on your peace of mind. Ask yourself whether you are committed to your relationship – whether you're ready to 'make old bones together'.

Perhaps you've already made 'old bones' together – an achievement that says a lot about the strength of your relationship. Over a long period you must both have changed, and in some ways become different people from the couple who initially got together. But growth and change carry on, and sometimes the stumbling block for a long-term relationship comes late in the day. I have several late middle-age female patients who, after a long and successful marriage, are starting to feel that their partners are holding them back. They've suddenly started calling themselves 'Ms' and are talking about moving to the city, perhaps embarking on further education or developing their careers. What's going on here is that, for one reason or another, these women have had occasion to review their lives and their priorities, and have found their partners wanting. Consider your own relationship – have you and your partner matured together, or grown apart? Do you need to review your priorities together?

Summing up

In this chapter we've covered a lot of ground, including aspects of developmental, personal and health psychology. Obviously we've only skimmed the surface of many issues, each of which could easily fill a book in its own right. The intention has been to get you thinking about your life, and about the different elements of it that make you happy or unhappy, including things you might not be consciously aware of. Before you can put things right you have to know what's wrong, and before you can restore equilibrium, you have to know the nature and cause of the imbalance. These principles hold true for your psychological health as much as for other aspects of the naturopathic triangle.

If this chapter seems to you to stray into territory you wouldn't normally think appropriate for a health book, then I'm pleased. Separating the psychological from the physical is misguided and misleading. It's important to see them both in context, but this is something that's increasingly rarely done in a conventional medical setting – again, highlighting the need for a doctor to fully understand a patient 'in context'. A life review of this sort helps you to do just that – to see things in context. By challenging your own priorities and assumptions, I hope that you can gain perspective and constructive insight into psychological issues, as well as health issues that may have psychological roots.

YOUR EMOTIONAL LIFESTYLE

- Do you have a happy work–life balance?

- Are you comfortable with yourself and with your friends and closest relatives?

- Which areas of your life would you like to improve?

CHAPTER 18

Rest and relaxation

When was the last time you proudly ticked 'Have a good long rest' off your 'to-do' list? Even if you do get enough rest and relaxation in your life, it's unlikely you consciously rate their importance as highly as a healthy diet, or trips to the gym. But as well as recharging our batteries in the most obvious physical sense – you can survive longer without food than without sleep, for instance – rest is the unsung hero of mental and emotional health. Lack of rest and relaxation leads to suppression of the immune system, headaches, poor appetite and fatigue, and so also to depression, irritability, lethargy, poor memory, diminished libido and slow and confused thinking. Improving both the quality and quantity of your rest and relaxation boosts all these areas, making you healthier, happier and sharper. But a lot of my patients need practical advice on how to overcome tension and insomnia, get more sleep, improve their relaxation skills, and generally make their life more restful.

Problems with sleep and relaxation can have physical causes, such as chronic pain or menopausal night sweats, but these do not affect everybody who has difficulty sleeping or resting. It's far more usual for stress to be the root cause. Modern lifestyles are filled with potential stressors, and almost everyone is exposed to some degree of it. What matters – as we've seen – is how you deal with it.

A core element of some Eastern philosophies, such as Zen Buddhism, is the need to let stress run off you. Letting it all just flow away is a valuable skill that everyone should apply to their own lives. It's important to distinguish between stressors that you can control or do something about, such as your workload or overscheduled diary, and those that you can't, like the behaviour of other people. Things you cannot control can 'clutter' your mind with negative and distracting thoughts that serve no useful purpose and simply cause tension. It's these that you must learn to let slide off you.

LETTING IT RUN OFF YOU

All religions teach some sort of acceptance or submission to the inevitable – to events or forces we cannot control. Whether we put our trust in God, seek the Buddhist 'middle way', or accept our karma on the Hindu wheel of life, we are letting uncontrollable events wash over us, while only seeking to take action where we can expect to be able to achieve some useful effect. Wisdom and enlightenment are highly prized in most Eastern religions, to raise us above the clamour and confusion of the emotional responses that are the causes of stress.

Stressful things we can do nothing about, like the noise of a busy road, or the behaviour of others, must not be allowed to get the better of us. Coping strategies such as refusing to be negatively affected by other people or finding practical solutions such as secondary glazing or heavy curtains must be carefully worked out. It is very important to retain an atmosphere of calm, and try to think of ways in which our reactions to stressors can be turned into something positive.

Four skills that can help you to achieve this are breathing, relaxation, meditation and sleeping. It may sound funny to hear breathing or sleeping described as skills, but in practice this is a useful way to think about them. As children we all knew how to do them, but as we grow up it is easy to acquire bad habits and 'unlearn' what was once instinctive. By 'retraining' in skills you once knew, and by learning new ones like meditation or relaxation, you can equip yourself with the tools you need to relieve stress and tension, clear your mind of distracting clutter and improve the quality and quantity of your rest and relaxation.

Breathing

One of the most common but least known effects of stress and anxiety is hyperventilation – breathing too quickly, or overbreathing. Although it can have other causes, it is usually linked to anxiety. Its origins are in the self-preserving human 'fight or flight' mechanism. Rapid breathing oxygenates the muscles in preparation for running or battle. The mechanism is very powerful, and rapid breathing can trigger the intense anxiety that helped our ancestors escape sabre-toothed tigers, but is not helpful in normal modern life.

Are you hyperventilating?

You might think this is a silly question – surely hyperventilators are people who suffer severe panic attacks and in their distress, gasp frantically for breath and have to breathe into brown paper bags? In extreme cases this might be true, but the symptoms of chronic hyperventilation are a lot more subtle. In one US study of people recovering from heart attacks, all were shallow breathers, never properly filling their lungs with clean air.

Stop a moment to watch the way you breathe (or ask someone else to observe you surreptitiously, so that you don't become self-conscious about your breathing), and ask yourself whether you've got any of the following symptoms:

- **Upper-chest breathing.** Breathing mostly with the upper chest and hardly at all with the diaphragm (the large sheet of muscle underneath your lungs). If your upper chest rises and falls a lot with each breath, but your stomach doesn't, then you're not breathing with your diaphragm.

- **Breathing faster than normal.** An average breathing rate at rest is 12 to 14 breaths a minute. Hyperventilators often lose the natural pause between breathing in and breathing out, and as a result may breathe up to twice as fast as normal.

- **Big breaths.** Taking a big breath before starting to speak, sighing deeply when pausing in speech and yawning a lot are signs of hyperventilation.

Some of these problems actually result from forgetting to breathe altogether. Tension can lead to literally 'holding one's breath' (unconsciously), which then leads to overcompensating again by hyperventilation.

Effects of hyperventilation   Scientists think that one reason why people hyperventilate is that in the short term it triggers the release of endorphins – brain chemicals similar to opiates, which elevate mood and relieve stress. The same chemicals are believed to be responsible for the 'runner's high' to which serious exercise nuts can become 'addicted'.

Unfortunately, the long-term effects of hyperventilation can be a lot more negative. Hyperventilators may experience a mixture of the following symptoms:

- Tiredness, due to the physiological effects and overuse of chest and neck muscles, which can also cause neck pain and tension headaches

- Rapid, sometimes irregular heartbeat

- Forgetfulness and irritability

- Tingling and numbness, which can mimic the effects of more serious conditions such as multiple sclerosis. Overbreathing causes excessive 'blowing off' of carbon dioxide via the lungs, which disturbs the body's biochemistry. This can account for some of the physical symptoms, such as tingling or palpitations

- Panic attacks, which can be seriously frightening, with feelings of difficulty breathing, a sense of impending doom and 'out of body' sensations.

Breathe easy   Once you've recognised the symptoms of hyperventilation, you can 'retrain' your breathing patterns. This takes practice and time – you need to perform the exercise below at least twice a day. However, the process itself is a good means of relaxation, and anyone can benefit from trying it out, whether they hyperventilate or not.

Lie on a bed or sit in a comfy chair with head and arm rests. Put one hand on your chest and one on your upper abdomen, so that you can feel them moving up and down as you breathe. Because you need to be completely relaxed all over, it may be a good idea to support your arms with cushions. Watching yourself in a mirror is another good way to keep tabs on your breathing.

Now you need to concentrate on breathing with the correct rhythm and timing. Start by clearing your lungs for action – take a small breath and let it out immediately, breathing all the way out, but slowly and without forcing. Then pause for two beats before breathing in again, draw in a new breath over a count of two beats, release it over a count of four beats, and pause again for two beats before drawing a new breath. Reffering to the second hand of a watch may help.

When you breathe in, your chest should move as little as possible – all the effort and movement should come from your diaphragm, so that your abdomen rises and falls with each breath. To start with you might need to take big breaths to be able to keep this rhythm. If so, take them slowly (one every 10 seconds, or six per minute). With practice, you should get better at using your diaphragm, and should try to take slightly smaller breaths, at a rate of about 10 to 12 per minute.

Your twice-daily practice sessions should help you to become aware of good and bad breathing habits, and the more you practise, the more time you'll spend breathing properly without thinking about it. At first, however, you'll have to monitor your breathing from time to time throughout the day, and keep a particular eye out for sighing, deep breathing/yawning and breath-holding before or during speech. You can improve your breathing while talking by reading aloud and at the same time concentrating on diaphragmatic breathing.

Retraining your breathing can be quite hard – you might like to consider consulting a specialised physiotherapist. But the long-term benefits will be worth it – more energy, fewer headaches, less tension, and a better reaction to stress.

Relaxation and meditation

It's hard to overstress the benefits of relaxation, especially in today's hectic world. But how many people do you know who actively take time out to relax

– to focus on the process of relaxation itself, rather than by watching TV or going to a bar? Not many, I'll bet, which is a shame, because doing a relaxation exercise for just a few minutes each day can change your life.

There are many different relaxation exercises and techniques you can try – below is one called the 'Relaxation Response', which I use with my patients. It's nice and simple, and accessible to anyone. You may notice similarities with the breathing technique outlined above. This is no coincidence – proper breathing is the foundation for most types of relaxation and meditation.

The Relaxation Response

You need to be comfortable and undisturbed for about 20 to 25 minutes, so settle down somewhere out of the way on a bed or comfy chair and make sure you have enough clothes/coverings to stay warm. Close your eyes and start to visualise tension draining out of your body. Feel your muscles loosen, starting at the feet and moving up to your face.

Concentrate on your breathing. Breathe through your nose and with your diaphragm. As you breathe out, say something to yourself (silently), any short word that helps clear your mind, like 'one', 'easy', 'relax' – I particularly recommend 'one' as it's not 'about' anything and so isn't too distracting. In order to relax, you need to focus solely on your chosen word, clearing your mind of all other thoughts. Distracting thoughts will occur – when they do, return to your word and focus only on it. Keep your breathing easy and as natural as you can.

The main problem for beginners (apart from inadvertently falling asleep!) is trying too hard. This can stop you from breathing naturally and make you hold your breath or breathe too deeply, leading to slight dizziness. It can also cause tension in areas such as the jaw or neck. Adopt a passive attitude, focus on your word and your breathing and let relaxation happen at its own pace.

This may sound contradictory – although you are trying to relax, you mustn't actually *try*! You're actively attempting to do something, but it's actually a passive thing that cannot be forced. This is why relaxation takes practice. Don't be put off if you're having trouble at first – the more you practise, the easier it will be to slip into the correct state.

Relax for about 15 to 20 minutes, and then start to focus on sensations other than your breathing and your word. If you're at home, you are very likely to fall asleep – which is no bad thing. Don't use an alarm clock to time yourself, as waiting for an alarm automatically causes stress! When you've finished, sit quietly with your eyes closed for a few minutes, and then with your eyes open. Stand up slowly.

Practise the Relaxation Response once or twice a day, but wait for two hours after a meal, since a full stomach and the digestion process seems to interfere with it. Try and do it at roughly the same time every day – that way you'll be more likely to get into the habit and less likely to skip a session. It can be done quietly at your desk or in a rest room, sitting or lying. When you start practising, don't let a day go by without doing it at least once daily. You are learning a very valuable tool that will prevent you from developing physical symptoms in stressful situations. It also feels really good.

The Relaxation Response 'resets' your breathing and thought rhythms, loosens tense muscles and relieves headaches. Successfully clearing your mind of all the 'butterfly' thoughts that normally occupy it, even if only for a few seconds, can have a profound effect on your peace of mind and stress levels for the whole day. Knowing that you have this skill to fall back on can be fortifying in itself, and if things do get hectic or stressful, a 10 to 15-minute break to practise the Relaxation Response can stop getting things from getting on top of you.

For those who suffer from insomnia, even for long periods, a relaxation technique practised on getting off to sleep and on waking can really work. Psychologists managing insomnia will certainly use relaxation techniques, which can help people slowly reduce their need for sleep-inducing medication.

An inner harmony

The Relaxation Response incorporates simplified forms of elements of meditation found in Buddhism, Hinduism, Christianity and many other religions and philosophies. There's calmness, breathing and a sort of mantra (a word or phrase that is chanted repetitively to help clear the mind of distractions and give a sense of peace). But the Relaxation Response falls short of more serious 'programmes' of meditation, because it isn't as all-embracing as them.

Personally, I'm in favour of wider-reaching systems of meditation and relaxation, for example if they form part of your religious beliefs and practices. As with dieting and exercise, relaxation and meditation shouldn't simply be 'stuck-on' things – they should become integral parts of your life, changing the way you approach life and therefore deal with stress.

Meditation is a way of unifying your self with a higher consciousness and helping to restore your inner harmony and equilibrium – and ultimately, achieving a greater peace of mind. Naturopathy works in a similar way, recognising a human need to tie together the physical and psychological with the spiritual.

MEN AND RELAXATION

Both men and women get stressed, but in my practice I find that women are much more open to doing something about it. Men don't seem willing to admit that stress could be a problem, and are uncomfortable about considering stress relief and relaxation techniques such as massage, hypnotherapy, t'ai chi, reiki or Bach Flower Remedies.

Yoga can be an ideal technique to learn. It has broad appeal and is also an excellent way to relax while getting into shape at the same time. So if you don't feel that acupuncture or aromatherapy are very 'you', or you know someone who needs to relax but doesn't know how, I advise yoga as a great route to relaxation. Of course, any form of exercise helps you to relax, generating endorphins and a healthful form of physical tiredness. But rather than high activity exercise such as squash or some other intensely competitive games, consider taking up something more rhythmical and steady – swimming, rowing or distance running, say – as part of your relaxation programme.

Sleep

You will spend around 25 years of your life asleep. It's the single most common human 'activity'. And although relatively little research has been done on sleep, despite its obvious importance, we do know that it is vital to your physical, physiological and psychological health.

Total sleep deprivation leads rapidly to mental and physical breakdown, followed by death. This is not, of course, a state many of us are likely to get into, but we regularly fail to get adequate sleep, and often damage the quality of what sleep we do get. In doing so we build up a sleep deficit – an amount of sleep that is 'owed' to our bodies – which generally gets paid off to some extent at weekends and on holidays. Until we've 'repaid' that deficit, however, it impairs our physical and mental abilities, leading to impaired performance at work, home and elsewhere (for instance, sleepiness is now responsible for more fatal accidents on the roads than alcohol or drugs).

So how much sleep do you really need? Well, there's no one-size-fits-all figure, but the answer is probably more than you're getting now. If you need an alarm clock to wake you in the morning, you're not getting enough sleep and you're building up a sleep deficit.

If you really want to find out how much sleep you need, take advantage of your next holiday period to experiment:

- Keep a notepad, pen and clock by your bed. Note down the time you turn off your light.

- Let yourself wake up naturally, without an alarm clock, and note down the time.

- Repeat this for as many days as possible – ideally at least a week.

For the first few days you'll probably sleep late, because you're paying off your accumulated sleep deficit. Eventually your sleeping time should even out. Leaving out the first few days, add up your total hours spent sleeping and divide by the number of nights – the result is your average sleep requirement.

Knowing how much sleep you *should* be getting is all very well, but most people end up going to bed too late to get the full amount. But you can at least improve the sleep you *are* getting by following a few simple tips:

- Make sure your bed, pillows, mattress and so on are comfortable – don't economise.

- Maintain a medium to cool temperature in your bedroom. Err on the side of coolness.

- Make sure your bedroom is quiet. If there is troublesome or disturbing noise outside, use earplugs or a radio tuned to 'white noise', the bit between radio stations intended to mask outside noise, which can mask other sounds.

- Make your bedroom a calm and peaceful place (see 'Unclutter your life', below). Try not to work, argue or do anything else that's stressful just before bedtime.

- Have curtains or blinds that block out all light – it can make a great difference to the quality of your sleep.

- Don't exercise late in the evening, as it will keep you awake and you need further time to 'unwind' from it. Allow at least two hours between exercise and sleeping, and preferably more.

- Limit your caffeine intake and don't drink anything containing caffeine after mid-afternoon. Also avoid alcohol, cigarettes and other drugs before bedtime – they interfere with the natural cycles you need to get the full benefit from your sleep.

- Avoid eating just before bedtime.

Overcoming insomnia

Insomnia is a serious consequence of stress, one that can lead to a vicious cycle. Lack of sleep is stressful in itself, impairs your performance so that life becomes more stressful and makes you less able to cope with stress. The result is worse insomnia.

To get out of this rut and stop draining your reserves of energy and health you need to tackle your problems at source – in other words, deal with the stressors in your life and the way you react to them. Obviously this would be a lot easier if you could get a decent night's sleep to start with, and the following 'Bathtime Relaxation' exercise should help you a great deal. It uses a gentle drop in body temperature – one of the cues your body and brain use to switch into sleep mode.

The idea of the exercise is to relax in the bath and then transfer to your bed with as little disruption as possible, so if there are things you need to do before you go to sleep – setting out your clothes for the next morning, locking doors and windows – get them out of the way before you begin. Also prepare your bed and bedroom: draw the curtains, set the alarm and put a hot water bottle in the bed if it's winter. Make sure no one's going to interrupt you.

Take several large towels into the bathroom, put them within easy reach of the tub and run a warm bath. Obviously it has to be a comfortable temperature (you'll be in it for around 20 minutes), so aim for warm – don't run it so hot that it's steaming. Make the bathroom atmosphere as soothing as possible – use dim lighting or candles (safely placed) and add bath salts, oils and so on to the water to soothe you. If you've got long hair, it might be an idea to tie it up or put on a bathing cap so that you don't have to bother drying it later.

Get comfortable in the bathtub and relax your whole body from the feet upwards. If you find it hard to relax, consider practising the Relaxation Response (see page 245). Combined with the warmth of the bath seeping into your muscles, this can make for a very soothing experience, but don't let yourself fall asleep at this stage – sleeping in a full bath is dangerous.

Caution: If you suffer from epilepsy, a heart condition or other serious health problems you need to exercise caution when bathing, and ensure that another household member knows that you're in the bath.

Lie in the bath relaxing for around 20 minutes, and then let the water out. (I do this with my toes so that I don't have to get up, which helps to keep me as relaxed as possible.) When the water has run out stay in the still hot bathtub (ideally you need a cast iron or steel bathtub – they absorb and then re-radiate heat well) and pull the towels on top of you, so that you are completely covered from head to foot. Being cocooned like this should help you to relax even more and it's safe to nod off at this point, although you don't want to wake up in a cold bathtub.

As soon as you start to feel cooler, wrap yourself snugly in the towels and slowly get out of the bath and eventually into your warm bed. Hopefully by now you'll be ready to nod off quickly, but if you still can't get to sleep try practising the Relaxation Response (see page 245) while lying in bed.

SIX WAYS TO DE-STRESS YOUR LIFE

1. **De-clutter**. Just as a cluttered mind can be stressful, dissipating your energy with 'butterfly' thoughts that distract you from your real goals, so a cluttered environment can be stressful. For instance, a work desk covered in bits of paper and half-done work doesn't simply reflect your stress – it helps to create it. Getting organised and clearing up clutter helps at every level. Finishing a backlog of nagging tasks and clearing your desk allows you to gain some focus and clearing the clutter from your environment can help to bring you peace of mind. Look around your house and ask yourself whether you've got too much stuff. Try clearing it away and see whether spending a few weeks living amidst a more minimalist aesthetic has a calming effect. This rule should particularly apply in your bedroom – keep work and other activities out, and reserve it exclusively for sleeping and being with your partner.

2. **Bring more light into your environment**. Do you live and work in dim light, under fluorescent lighting, surrounded by busy wallpaper or without a window or a view? See if you can brighten things up with a lick of bright or light paint, or by clearing obstructions away from sources of natural light and with plants or flowers. Sunlight in particular affects our mood and some people become depressed or listless when the days shorten towards winter. This condition, called seasonal affective disorder (SAD), occurs when a lack of exposure to sunlight depresses melatonin production in the brain, leading to a depressed mood. If you have SAD, make a real effort to get out into daylight, especially early in the morning. Being out in natural daylight, even on a dull day, can make a real difference. So try hard to make the effort to go for a morning walk, maybe as part of your journey to work. If this is impractical, you could consider a light box (see Resources).

3. **Get into the countryside**. I know I'm always extolling the virtues of getting out of town, but if you live in a big city it's easy to forget just how important the calming, regenerative atmosphere of more natural surroundings can be. Free time spent walking in woods, by the coast or even in a city park is time well spent.

4. **Dew walking**. Naturopathy stresses using all your senses, especially the more neglected ones like touch. During late spring and summer, if you have access to a garden or anywhere with a patch of grass, try taking off your shoes and socks and walking barefoot on the grass in the early morning or evening. The feel of the cool dew and wet grass on your bare feet is an enlivening experience. It may sound silly, but try it – you'll be surprised how relaxing and enjoyable it is. In fact, it's a great way to clear a foggy head when you get up in the morning and very pleasant when the dew comes down on a summer evening and the shadows stretch across the garden.

5. **Stroke an animal**. Anyone with a pet will tell you what a rewarding experience it is to interact with an animal. Stroking a dog, cat, horse or any other animal stimulates all your senses, while the unconditional love of a pet, and the affection and responsibility you return to it, make good 'soul food'. Animals can be excellent therapists, and many people feel much better after a chat with their dog or cat.

6. **Listen to music**. Again, this might seem obvious, but the calming effects of music are underestimated. The right sort of music can help you to contemplate, relax and take your mind off other things. Bach and Vivaldi are special favourites of mine. Try listening to loads of different kinds of music, from jazz to Gregorian chant and the latest chart hits.

CHAPTER 19

Peace of mind

M any people end up in my clinic because they're reassessing their priorities. The threat of illhealth, anxieties about imminent retirement, or the realisation that success in business isn't going to bring happiness – any of these can cause someone to reassess their values and realise they need to make lifestyle changes. Hopefully some of what you have read so far has made you take stock of your life too. Are you happy with your work–life balance, for example? Or have you identified facets of your personality and abilities that you are not expressing or exploring fully enough? Are you fully exploiting your creative potential? To return to one of the questions in Chapter 1 – if the world was to end today, would you feel your time had been well spent?

When evaluating psychological wellbeing I am interested in how much creativity and fun you have in your life, whether you have any 'unfinished business', how assertive you are in certain situations, how you approach responsibility and manage your time, and how well your social network is functioning. So, as you see, there's a lot more to it than simply looking for signs of stress and depression.

Creativity

I have treated numerous people with problems they find hard to articulate. They might be doing well in their career, with all the outward trappings of a successful life, but cannot shake off a lingering sense of malaise. When we get to the root of their problem, there is very often a deeply entrenched sense of frustration at stifled creativity. They may talk longingly about earlier times, usually before they were set on their career path, when they got more of a chance to express themselves through music, art or dance, for example. Every one of us has a creative side, which brings self-fulfilment and boosts psychological health. But in my experience, many people pay too little attention to this side of themselves.

Are there periods of your life you look back on with particular fondness or times when you felt particularly excited and engaged by what you were doing? It doesn't matter how far back you have to go, or how trivial or brief it seems with hindsight, so long as you can say about it, 'This was something that made me feel really good!'

Alternatively, think about what you would be doing in an 'ideal scenario' – that is, if you could be doing any career or pursuit at all. Although the fantasy situation may be extreme, its theme may be accessible. For instance, your ideal scenario might be that you'd like to be a movie star – while stardom might not be feasible, anyone can at least try learning the craft of acting and enjoying the social scene and 'buzz' that surrounds a production.

Express yourself

But not everyone is interested in acting, writing, music or painting. Remember – anything that allows you to express yourself can be creative, whether it's sport, travelling, dance, interior decoration, carpentry, building models or decorating a doll's house, arranging parties, gardening, visiting museums, or working with children. And of course you don't have to limit yourself to just one interest.

Once you've identified the thing or things that you really feel enthusiastic about, you need to start your research. One way of doing this is by joining a group of people who share your interests. You could look into adult education classes, volunteer groups, hobby associations, gyms, graduate associations and the like. You might be surprised at how many 'extracurricular' opportunities there are around.

Or you could always take charge yourself and organise activities with your friends or other like-minded people. Start up your own Sunday soccer league, tennis tournament, walking group or reading club. Put on a play starring your family. The possibilities are endless.

Not all creative pastimes have to be engineered. Watch children playing and you'll see how creative and imaginative they are. I am a great advocate of horsing around – out of doors, if possible. Playing is both invigorating and relaxing, in that it clears the mind of stressful thoughts and is a powerful tool for focusing on the world of the immediate – sensation, activity and interaction in the here and now. Obviously it's a lot easier to horse around if you've got kids, or at least a dog or a garden swing, but the principle applies in a more general sense – try to see the funnier side of life more often, to relax and not take things too seriously.

Unfinished business

Developing a new approach to life that allows you to find peace of mind means that you'll need to level with any emotional baggage you're carrying, and free yourself from your emotional anchors. But how best to deal with this 'unfinished business'?

Unfinished business can also stem from physical diseases or problems that linger on in people who won't 'let go' of them. Naturopaths call this 'hanging on to your condition'. It can involve a kind of learned dependency, in which the person learns to depend on the support, care and attention they receive when they've been unwell – so they tend to continue in this role. Therapist dependency, where a patient finds it very hard not to keep going back for the attention and ministrations of therapists, can also be a problem. When something is playing an important psychological role in your life, even a negative one, it can be hard to let go. This is why unfinished business can be difficult to resolve.

You can only 'let go' of an issue if you have truly made your peace with it. This is why psychologists talk about 'closure' – and unless you have a sense of having closed an issue you will not truly be able to move on. If something is bugging you – anxiety about your health, unresolved grief, regret – to the extent that it enters your thoughts frequently, affects your outlook or the way you live, then it is time for you to address this issue.

But first you have to admit to what's bothering you, in a safe and supportive environment. Doing this in a literal, physical sense can sometimes be a good idea. For example, you could write down your issue and how you feel about it. Close friends can make excellent substitutes for therapists, but often it's preferable and actually much easier to discuss a difficult subject with a professional who brings the benefits of their training and experience, especially when you know that confidentiality is guaranteed. A comfortable and appropriate professional relationship is invaluable and undoubtedly this is one reason why patients often reveal hidden feelings, fears and burdens to me, and feel less inhibited about showing their true emotions.

Once you've identified the issues you need to deal with, try looking at them from a more objective viewpoint. To assess problems without being clouded by emotion, break them down into their elements or component parts, and consider each one individually. Are there practical solutions to some of the problems, or are they issues over which you have no control? 'Change what you can, accept what you can't' is a useful guide.

Assertiveness

Twenty-first-century living is a stressful business, and how we respond to it is a huge part of how we live our lives. But it isn't always easy to understand the patterns of stress in our lives: the causes and effects of stress form a complex tangle of interactions, feedbacks and vicious circles.

For instance, if you take on too much work, inevitably you won't get it all done. This may lead to a sense of failure and inferiority, causing low self-esteem and depression. These in turn prevent you from being as effective or efficient in your job, so that you get even less done and feel even worse – and more stressed.

Paradoxically, at the same time that you're getting less done, you may be taking on more, because low self-esteem makes people very bad at saying 'no'. If you're feeling like this, when your boss at work says he needs you to write his report for him and your colleague asks if you'll cover her afternoon meetings, you may simply nod meekly and acquiesce rather than risk having a confrontation. In short, you lack assertiveness. Other signs may be problems accepting or giving compliments, and an inability to express frustrations or problems with partners, friends or colleagues.

Obviously, employers reward those with 'can-do' attitudes, and ambitious employees want to 'step up to the plate' to show they're worth promoting.

However, there's a big difference between ambition and a willingness to get stuck in, on the one hand, and fear of setting reasonable limits on the other. If you've already got too much on your plate, you won't be doing anyone (and least of all yourself) any favours by taking on more, because in the long run, all your work will suffer.

Equally, ducking conflicts or avoiding difficult discussions with friends, partners and colleagues may sound like a sensible policy in the short term, but bottling problems up leads to festering resentments and poisoned relationships.

Assertive – or aggressive?

Some people confuse assertiveness with aggression. Saying 'no' to your boss or expressing frustration with a partner might sound a bit like aggressive behaviour, but there's a difference. Assertiveness involves expressing yourself directly, honestly and openly while still respecting the feelings, opinions and rights of other people. Aggression is being assertive at the expense of others, without respecting them – and if you find yourself (or others) accusing or insulting the other person, being pushy, 'letting rip', sneering or name-calling, you'll see how different this approach is from being assertive. But the demarcation between the two can seem subtle, and this is one reason why many people are shy of being more assertive.

Learning to become truly assertive has many benefits. For starters, you can avoid taking on extra burdens and stresses, thus lightening your load and making you better able to cope with the work you already have. In a more general way it will boost your self-esteem and make you a more effective person. Other people will respect you more, as your ability to communicate with them improves and you grow to respect yourself more.

How to be more assertive

- Be honest, direct and firm. Don't be embarrassed to have an opinion or make a demand. You have as much right as anyone else. Don't disown or undermine your opinions or feelings.

- Use the word 'no' in response to unreasonable demands, and be clear and firm about it. Don't cave in or prevaricate.

- Don't be afraid to ask for an explanation from a superior or colleague if asked to do something unreasonable.

- Be polite at all times, but don't apologise or make excuses for saying no or being assertive when you feel you're in the right.

- Use calm but assertive body language – stand up straight; face people front on and maintain eye contact; maintain a comfortable distance from people.

- Don't be rushed into responses.

- When making statements, especially about your feelings, talk about yourself rather than criticise the other person. Use the word 'I' rather than 'you' (which is more aggressive).

- Don't raise your voice or get angry. Don't accuse, or be insulting or pushy.

- Accept compliments graciously. Give compliments, but only honestly, and don't feel obliged to return a compliment.

- Don't duck difficult issues – if you feel unhappy about something, say so.

- Give yourself due credit and let others know about your achievements.

Being in control

As we saw in Chapter 17, one of the factors that influences your perception of, and response to, stress is your sense of control – that is, the degree of control you feel you have over a stressful situation. Experiments show that people deal much better with stress when they feel more in control.

Responsibility = control

In your day-to-day life, being in control is tied up with other issues like assertiveness and self-esteem. Part of being more assertive involves taking responsibility – for your actions and their consequences, and for your feelings and opinions.

Taking control and being responsible applies to your mental and physical health. If you relinquish control over issues in your life such as healthcare, diet or working hours, not only do they become more stressful as a result, but there is also less you can do when things go wrong.

Chronic illness can be a good example of this principle. Suppose that you suffer from asthma. If you simply regard yourself as a passive victim, whose only option is to follow doctor's orders and take ever-increasing doses of medication without question, then your condition is not under your control. The chances of improvement will be low and your illness will become an increasing source of stress.

Alternatively, you could take responsibility for your own healthcare. If you learn what you can about asthma, take steps to reduce your exposure to triggers and exacerbating factors, work to reduce your dependence on medication and challenge your doctor to provide a more holistic approach to asthma management, you will be in control of your condition. Studies show that patients with this approach to their condition suffer less illness.

Taking responsibility is also an important element in achieving closure of unfinished business (see above). Long-nurtured grievances – perhaps old hurts or disappointments that you blame on someone else – can be hard to let to go of unless you take responsibility for past actions as well as present or future ones. If you can admit that you too bear responsibility for the unfinished business, you can then try to make your peace with yourself and move on.

Time management

A lot of the advice in this book revolves around the need to make more time for one activity or another, whether it be exercise, meditation, cooking fresh meals or playing with your kids. This may seem paradoxical, given that pressures on your time are a major cause of the stress that such activities are intended to help relieve.

If pressures on your time are indeed a source of stress, the question is 'Why?' The obvious answer is that too many people are demanding too much of you – usually at work, where you're probably being asked to do more and more in the same amount of time. The other possible reason is that you're not using your time efficiently and/or effectively, wasting too much of it on minor tasks and unproductive activities. In both cases you might benefit from adopting some time management skills that can help you to rationalise and prioritise your workload, and focus your efforts.

THE 80:20 RULE: THE PARETO PRINCIPLE

Studies show that people typically generate 80 per cent of results from 20 per cent of their effort. The other 80 per cent of their efforts are unfocused and wasteful, and contribute just 20 per cent of results. Although the actual ratio may vary from person to person, this principle – known as the Pareto Principle – remains the same. The purpose of time management systems is to change this ratio and increase the productive proportion of your time, getting the most out of inevitably limited resources.

Using your time well

This is a health manual, not a management or business self-help guide, so I won't go into lengthy detail about the particulars of time management systems. They come in all shapes and sizes, and it doesn't really matter which one you follow anyway, as long as it encourages you to reflect on your use of time – to step back from being in the midst of your life and see it in perspective, and in focus. (A panoramic shot, if you like.) Most of the systems, however, have elements or stages in common, and these are relevant not just from the point of view of work, employers and so on, but also for increasing your efficiency and efficacy in all walks of life.

A typical first step in a time management system is to make a proper analysis of how you spend your time, so that you can see where it's being wasted and where it's being used productively. Because it can be hard to get an objective picture of something like this, a technique called 'costing' is often used. This is where you work out what your time is worth per hour, and then use this figure to cost your various activities. Costing allows you to recast ambiguous statements – such as 'I'm wasting too much time making to-do lists' – in concrete terms – 'I wasted £2300 of my time last year on making to-do lists.'

Analysing your time usage is a valuable technique for all areas of your life, not just work. Look at how long you spend working versus other activities, using costing and possibly an activity log (like a detailed diary) to put concrete figures to each category. You might discover, for instance, that the imbalance between work and play in your life is far greater than you realised.

Dreams and aspirations

A second step in many time management programmes is to determine what your priorities are, and whether you are working accordingly. By combining this step with step one (analysing your time usage) you can get a clear picture of how much of your time is devoted to your priorities, and how much you might be frittering away on things that don't really matter to you. Again, this is a technique that can be applied to every aspect of your life – management and motivation gurus call it 'personal goal setting'.

Personal goal setting involves writing down goals for each of the main areas of your life, arranging them in order of priority and then breaking them down into 'sub-goals' – the intermediate stages you'll need to reach on the way to attaining your lifetime goals. For instance, if your lifetime goal in the area of 'physical health' is 'to remain mobile and independent into my eighties', one of your sub-goals might be 'to run a half-marathon at age 55'. You then break down the sub-goals into more immediate, short-term goals, until you arrive at what is essentially a road map for achieving your lifetime goals. Headings under which you might consider setting goals include: career, family, financial, health, creativity, travel and community.

The various goals should be positive and ambitious without being unrealistic. You should try to avoid setting goals that are not really within your control – for instance, 'write a novel and submit it to publishers' is better than 'write a novel that is immediately snapped up by a publisher and becomes a bestseller'.

Breaking down your lifetime goals into intermediate and short-term goals gives you something manageable and realistic to aim at. Having a concrete, practical goal means you are less likely to be diverted or discouraged, while achieving goals is good for your self-esteem, confidence and motivation. It also makes it much easier to monitor your progress.

This applies at all levels, from the annual report you have to write on top of your weekly workload, to your ultimate ambition to become a concert-level pianist. One of the secrets of successful people is that they break down big tasks into smaller chunks, which are inherently more manageable and less stressful, helping them to stay cool, calm and collected and achieve ambitious overall goals. The same strategy can be used to help you achieve a more active lifestyle with a rounded exercise programme and a better diet incorporating varied and healthy foods.

Social roots: be like a tree

Naturopathy teaches us to look at healing as a continuous process, providing us with a sort of health insurance for the future. The best way to build up mental and emotional reserves that will protect you against future challenges and crises is to 'think like a tree'. A tree can't control future conditions – and it can't escape what the weather and other outside forces will do to it. But it can put down the longest, deepest, strongest roots possible so that it is firmly embedded in the soil and can draw resources from a wide area. If you're to weather the storms of the future well, you'll need to put firm roots down within your social environment: your family, friends and community.

Studies show that having a strong social network, with lots of friends and close ties to your community, boosts your immune system, extends your life-span, decreases any bouts of ill health and improves your recovery from illness.

But this is only one side of having lots of people in your life. Friends can also be demanding and difficult – a source of stress. Psychologists identify a number of factors that determine whether your friends are a help or a hindrance:

- Friends who give too little support obviously aren't very good friends, but sometimes friends can give too much support, crowding you or making you dependent and undermining your self-esteem.

- Friends who give the wrong kind of support can boost stress levels – you might be looking for just 'tea and sympathy', but your friend might think that practical solutions or 'tough love' are what you really need.

- Friends who are stuck in a rut or not adaptable themselves may not support you when you try to make changes, such as kicking bad health habits like smoking or starting a new career. The closer you are to your friends (the denser your social network, in technical terms), the more likely this is to be a problem.

When you look at the list above, would you regard yourself as a good friend and source of support to your friends? Given how important friends are to all aspects of your health, it's really important to value them and invest in your social network. Don't let friendships die away through lack of effort or pressures of work. Cultivate good 'friendship habits' – show your appreciation of your friends regularly, become a good listener, give more hugs.

Getting involved

Remember to look outward: do things for the benefit of others, such as getting involved with the community through charity or volunteer work. During the 1980s, classic studies by the psychologist Julius Segal showed that those coping with the aftermath of terrible traumas, such as Holocaust survivors, refugees and freed hostages, had much better outcomes when they got involved with helping others. By showing compassion, they helped to heal themselves.

Looking outwards in this way helps people to cope with everyday stress, too. It makes them better at looking for solutions instead of apportioning blame, helps them to see both sides of an argument and not take things too personally, and gives them a better sense of perspective and priorities. It's the social equivalent of a tree putting down strong roots and growing together with other trees to make a forest – a healthily interrelated, living community.

Getting outside help

You may have tried a number of ways to feel more connected, more in control, more assertive and so on, but still feel distressed, lonely, angry or depressed. Be aware that you're not alone. The World Health Organization has found that depression is on the rise worldwide. More importantly, be assured that a good therapist can help set you back on track, kick-starting your own ability to get out of an emotional rut, or helping you weather a longer-term trauma. But there's a lot of confusion about the different types of mental health professionals, particularly psychotherapists, psychologists, psychiatrists and psychoanalysts.

Mental health professionals: which is which?

Psychotherapists A psychotherapist is anyone who practises a form of psychotherapy – that is, listening to and discussing problems or issues using a certain psychological approach or mixture of approaches. Some forms of psychotherapy involve hypnosis, looking closely at clients' behaviour patterns, or even using art, storytelling, music, humour or movement. A psychotherapist should be trained in one or more approaches, as well as have more general training in psychology, and should be registered with an accepted body. But there's no legal requirement for this, so in fact anyone can call themselves a psychotherapist.

Psychoanalysts are psychotherapists who follow the Freudian model, where the client uses free association, dream interpretation and other techniques to explore anxieties, conflicts, repressed desires and so on.

Psychologists A psychologist is anyone who has studied psychology. In the context of treatment, however, it usually means a clinical psychologist – someone who has trained and qualified in psychology and evaluates and monitors people with emotional health problems. Although they are not doctors, which usually means they're not allowed to prescribe drugs, they often practise forms of psychotherapy. So a psychotherapist could also be a psychologist.

Psychiatrists A psychiatrist is a medical doctor who has trained and qualified in the specialist field of psychiatry – the medical treatment of mental illness. They are allowed to prescribe drugs, but many also practise some form of psychotherapy.

When to see a therapist

As you may have already discovered, a lot of people believe that mental problems aren't 'real' problems, and that you should either ignore them or sort them out yourself – the 'stiff upper lip'/'pull up your socks' approach. Other people point out that a course of therapy is usually quite expensive, and that if you need to talk things over with someone you should use your friends or family. So when is it worthwhile to see a therapist?

You should certainly see a therapist if you are suffering from conditions such as depression, obsessive-compulsive disorder or a phobia. These problems are often successfully treated with drugs. But drugs should not be the only answer – and some people don't respond well to them, while others develop too many side effects. Psychotherapy in combination with drugs is almost always more effective than drugs on their own, partly because through therapy a patient can learn skills, techniques and insights that will help them in the future.

Therapists are also useful if you're having sexual or relationship difficulties, or any other problems that you might find hard to discuss with friends or family. Increasingly, psychotherapy is being sought by people who don't necessarily have problems but want to take advantage of the power of psychology to make changes in their personal or professional life. In such cases a psychotherapist can be a sort of teacher on the one hand, and a useful catalyst for change on the other.

In any case, whatever the form of the therapy, the vital thing is that it works for you. How will you know? Because after several sessions, you will be feeling better about yourself, less down, energised and ready to get on with your life.

Types of psychotherapy

Since Sigmund Freud started the ball rolling with psychoanalysis at the start of the twentieth century, psychological theories have sprouted like mushrooms, bringing with them a host of ways to apply his theories, and those of his successors, through therapy. As a result there are literally hundreds of types and sub-types of psychotherapy, but most of them fall into one of a few groups.

Humanistic Many psychotherapists today use a more 'people-friendly' approach based on what are called humanistic theories, which stress personal happiness and self-fulfilment as well as personal responsibility. They look less at the past and more at the present.

Cognitive-behavioural Cognitive-behavioural therapy (CBT) is a very popular form of therapy for the treatment of depression. A course of CBT tends to be short (typically, 10 hour-long sessions), practical and effective, teaching the client useful psychological habits and skills that can be used long after the therapy is over.

CBT focuses on identifying and then changing the thoughts and behaviours that cause and reinforce problems such as depression. For instance, a therapist and client together might identify how the client reacts to normal events in an abnormally negative way. Suppose you dropped a bottle of milk – the normal way to respond might be to think, 'Oh, it was slippery.' If you were depressed you might think, 'I can't do anything right, I'm a failure.' The CBT approach here would be to help you see how distorted your thinking has become, and to make a conscious effort to substitute normal thoughts for negative ones.

The right therapy – and therapist – for you

The combination of a reassuring person with something to teach (the therapist) and a convincing theory (the type of therapy) gives the client a way to understand and explore problems and offers hope of overcoming them. The therapy process itself then tends to follow a similar pattern – client and therapist together gain insights into the problem, figure out a plan of action and work on it. This pattern holds true for other forms of counselling, such as that offered by a vicar or rabbi.

In fact, the therapist is usually more important in determining outcome than the kind of therapy you go for. What matters in particular is the relationship between client and therapist. Having said that, people will be drawn to a style of therapy they feel comfortable with. So the 'right' type of therapy is something quite personal and individual. Finding the right therapy-therapist combination for you is a matter of personal taste and, possibly, experimentation, although this is obviously not an option for many people.

Still, if you don't 'click' with your therapist, your therapy may not be as effective, so it's worthwhile viewing the first session of a course of therapy as a trial session.

While you are thinking about how best to get your emotional needs met with a therapist, I would advise that you see your doctor, who holds a responsibility for your care and is in a very good position to advise you. However, if you find yourself being prescribed drugs after a very short consultation, and you feel uncomfortable with this approach, say so or see another doctor with whom you feel comfortable. Alternatively, you can go and see a therapist privately – there are thousands to choose from. Find one in your area from private hospitals, your local health authority or even the Yellow Pages. You will need to check their membership of their professional body and their qualifications, and try to get some idea of how many sessions you may need. Therapy can be expensive.

- To get a head start on finding a therapist who suits you, see if you can get personal recommendations/descriptions, either from friends who might have seen a therapist or from your healthcare professionals.

- Remember that in some places, loose licensing regulations mean that almost anyone may be able to set themselves up as a therapist. Only go to a therapist who is registered by their professional body and carries insurance.

Summing up

I don't pretend to have a monopoly on wisdom or the answers to all of life's riddles. Apropos of mental health and finding the best way to organise your life, my advice is based on the lessons I have learned from my patients. Many of them encounter pain and problems, regrets or unhappiness; often those who seem outwardly most successful are those with the most loneliness and frustration. Together we have worked towards the various solutions and approaches outlined above, which I hope add up to at least a partial recipe for greater peace of mind, now and in the future.

PART **5**

Total Health

CHAPTER 20

Look forward

We go to our doctors for advice when we are unwell, or worried that something may be wrong. My patients are no different. This book is peppered with examples from my casenotes of people who have suffered from migraine, menstrual problems, allergies, IBS, back pain – all the modern-day ailments that make up a typical GP's workload. Even in this enlightened age of health education, when we are aware of the need to stay well in order to avoid the pitfalls of 'too much of a good thing', few of us ask for advice on maintaining or restoring our equilibrium. We do not ask how to keep our blood pressure at the healthy measurement it is today. We only begin to worry when we see it start to climb. A lot of us do not even consider how we will keep our weight where we like it. We just look for advice on getting it back to normal once the pounds are beginning to pile on.

But even if you started reading this book because you wanted to restore your blood pressure to a healthy level, shift a few excess pounds, or to get to the bottom of a mysterious suspected allergy, I hope that by now you will have realised that by redressing the balance in your lifestyle, you will not only help yourself to solve any current ailments, but will also prevent new ones from arising in the future.

Of course, many of these problems may not become apparent for many years to come. Arthritis, cancer, heart disease and diabetes are all more prevalent among the older generation – and it is often hard for us to look into the future and imagine how we will feel 20, 30, or 40 years down the line, if we succumb to one of these illnesses. Will we say, 'Hindsight is a wonderful thing', or 'Why didn't I hold on to my health while I had it?'

Well, hindsight is a wonderful thing. And, because of what we have learned from it, it enables us to improve our health – if we are prepared to make the necessary changes.

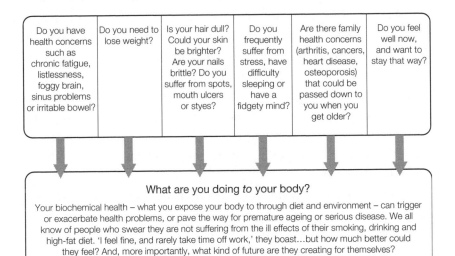

| Do you have health concerns such as chronic fatigue, listlessness, foggy brain, sinus problems or irritable bowel? | Do you need to lose weight? | Is your hair dull? Could your skin be brighter? Are your nails brittle? Do you suffer from spots, mouth ulcers or styes? | Do you frequently suffer from stress, have difficulty sleeping or have a fidgety mind? | Are there family health concerns (arthritis, cancers, heart disease, osteoporosis) that could be passed down to you when you get older? | Do you feel well now, and want to stay that way? |

What are you doing *to* your body?

Your biochemical health – what you expose your body to through diet and environment – can trigger or exacerbate health problems, or pave the way for premature ageing or serious disease. We all know of people who swear they are not suffering from the ill effects of their smoking, drinking and high-fat diet. 'I feel fine, and rarely take time off work,' they boast…but how much better could they feel? And, more importantly, what kind of future are they creating for themselves?

What are you doing *with* your body?

Keeping physically fit is, as we all know, one way to stabilise your weight and fend off disease. Your risk of cancer, heart disease and osteoporosis goes down if you take regular exercise. Exercise also has a calming effect on the mind, reducing your chances of succumbing to stress-related symptoms such as migraine and IBS. When your body copes well with stress, you are likely to stick to a healthy diet, and to use nutrients efficiently, thus keeping brittle nails, dry hair and dull skin at bay. You will sleep well, and find it easier to relax.

How's your state of mind?

Emotional health is vital, helping us cope with the stress that's the root of so much ill-health, and keeping us happy, connected and creative. Mind and body are intimately connected. If we're biochemically and physically healthy, we'll be giving our mental and emotional health a huge boost; and if we're mentally balanced and motivated, we're a lot more likely to kick (or never take up) bad habits such as smoking and binge drinking, and decide to live as long, active and healthy a life as we can.

Putting the health triangle into practice

Age of enlightenment

So, let's assume you are healthy now – and you want to remain this way. Early on in this book I was rather gloomily commenting on the fact that we are all living much longer these days – but that, sadly, a long old age often means many years of failing health. This, however, is far from inevitable. In fact, we are already beginning to see a change in the health of the elderly, and figures show that disability rates are falling as the effects of better healthcare, lifestyles and diets kick in. And as there are now far more people over 70 than there are kids under 15, that's all to the good. By the time today's fortysome-things reach their sixties, they will be in the majority. And, when we get there, the last thing we will want to be called is 'third age' or 'the grey popu-lation'. These terms make me think back to when I was a small child: I remember asking my mother why every woman over the age of 60 seemed to have the same curly grey perm. I think we should hold on to our individ-uality into our dotage.

But how well any of us will age is determined by a number of factors. If you have watched older relatives die prematurely or lead uncomfortable and limited lives in old age because of problems like arthritis, osteoporosis or diabetes, you may fear it is in your genes to succumb to the same fate. In fact, these prematurely ageing conditions may well be in your genes, although it is not your fate to succumb to them. There may be an inherited tendency towards some conditions, but to what extent that tendency is expressed can often be curbed by a healthy, consciously preventive lifestyle. The purpose of this book has been to highlight the ways in which you can take control of your health and wellbeing . . . and we do have a good deal of control over how we age – we just have to make the effort!

A patient recently phoned my secretary bemoaning the fact that it was so hard having to stick to the healthy regime I'd prescribed for her. In fact, it was a very mild plan designed to get her going in the right direction, and unfortunately I could not suggest a shortcut. To achieve results, changes do have to be made. Tellingly, when I saw her a couple of weeks later, she had cheered up no end as she was already feeling better and losing weight.

Of course, ageing is not just something that starts to happen to you when you reach the age of 50. It's a gradual but inevitable process that actually began from the moment you reached adult maturity, which is in your early twenties. The earlier you start to take the right steps in terms of your health and the way you live, the better your prospects for a vigorous, active and rewarding old age. In other words, ageing shouldn't only matter to the elderly – it's an important issue for us all. This is part of what I meant when I talked about building up reserves of health in earlier chapters.

NOT OVER THE HILL

To those born in the 1930s or 1940s, 60 was always seen as elderly, and 70 was when you expected to die (you'd had your 'three score years and ten'). Nowadays I tell patients all the time that 50 is the new 40, and 70 is the new 50. You're definitely not over the hill at this age – so don't let anyone make you think you are. Sadly, a lot of older people believe that their age is responsible for their health problems, and they do not insist on a thorough examination from their GP. I recently saw a lovely lady in her eighties, Elsa, who was suffering from infuriating and embarrassing vulval irritation. Her GP had not examined her, explaining that her symptoms were due to ageing – even though vulval cancer is something that tends to affect post-menopausal and elderly women almost exclusively. And having had her problem dismissed, Elsa was understandably reluctant to go back for more of the same! She needed to be examined and treated with care and respected. I had to build up her confidence and get her back into the medical system for the further tests she needed.

None of us should have to accept that, because of our age, our problems are irreversible and do not therefore warrant good medical care.

Your biochemical and physical health are, of course, crucial to the individual ageing process. But psychological health is absolutely vital. If we stay mentally fit as we age, we'll remain motivated to remain fit in every way.

Today, older people are always being exhorted to see their more mature years as a time of opportunities, and this is a healthy, positive approach to take. The trouble is that many people cannot reconcile such positive messages with their own anxieties and doubts. As I have discussed elsewhere in this book, a lot of people are stressed by identity and relationship worries, or maybe feeling lonely or financially insecure.

As they lose confidence in their abilities and appearance the effects can trigger a negative spiral. Loss of self-confidence leads to loss of self-esteem. Loss of self-esteem can lead in turn to physical, mental and social withdrawal. The less physical, mental and social effort they make, however, the more likely they are to fulfil their own predictions because with age the rule is 'use it or lose it'.

The botox issue

Personal problems of self-esteem can be exacerbated by the attitudes of society at large. We shouldn't underestimate the power of our very youth-oriented Western culture in fuelling feelings of inadequacy amongst older people. When botox injections and facelifts become run-of-the-mill and hair-dye sales soar into the stratosphere, we know we're living in a time of obsession with youth and appearance. To age gracefully, the best thing to do is simply to go on pursuing your own course of healthy eating, thinking and exercising. Letting the advertising and magazine articles get to you will simply add to any feelings of anxiety or low self-esteem.

But some people do succumb. I have had patients who have given up all forms of exercise because they're worried that they look silly wearing a tracksuit – and then they're upset because they really have got out of shape.

One of my patients, Olivia, had exactly this problem. At 50, Olivia felt slow, sluggish and unattractive. She had gained a lot of weight and seemed unable to shift it despite the low-fat diet she'd adopted. The most obvious thing to boost her weight loss would have been to take some exercise. But because of her poor self-esteem and body image, she didn't want to be seen in sports clothes. In the past, she'd played tennis in doubles with her husband. Now she refused to do this as she feared she'd look silly in her tennis skirt. He was starting to think she was no longer very much fun and I could see that the whole issue was starting to impinge on their relationship.

I persuaded Olivia to take a few one-to-one sessions with a personal trainer, and also to start walking regularly. Within four months she was down from 17 stone to 14 stone and feeling much jollier! She started playing tennis again (in joggers!) and this delighted her husband, who really hadn't been able to understand why she'd become so withdrawn.

Weight is an important issue as we age, but I am constantly telling patients it's even more important to consider the muscle to fat ratio. If one were to scan the thigh muscle of a 30-year-old it would be significantly greater than that of a 60-year-old, so aiming to maintain muscle bulk with an active life is crucial. We put the words 'old and frail' together because that is what happens to the body if we do not continue to work at fitness. Older people must work harder to retain their musculature than younger people, making exercise more important rather than something to be given up!

Think yourself young

Most of us, whatever our age, have had the experience of going into a room and wondering what we went in for. Words and names will elude us too. As we get older, we may worry that this is a sign of impending Alzheimer's. It's not! It's the same as it ever was – a sign of a busy and very active mind. Jean, a patient in her sixties, became very concerned that she was no longer 'on the ball' – but that was hardly surprising when I went over her history with her. She wasn't sleeping at all well because her mind was doing somersaults worrying about one of her grown-up daughters, who had anorexia. We are supposed to get older and wiser, but that doesn't stop us worrying as much as ever.

But thinking negatively about our mental condition, or what others might think, is detrimental. It's far better to embrace new intellectual and social challenges, and get on with the business of keeping our brains fit. Just as with physical exercise, doing this once or twice will get us 'hooked', and we'll soon find brainwork of all kinds fun.

Moira was 80 when she discovered her niche. After years of drudgery in a dreary administrative job, she took up art – something she'd adored as a child. She is now a member of an artist's group, with serious collectors interested in her work. Her life has been revolutionised at an age when so many negative-thinking people are deciding to throw in the towel.

Give your brain a workout

Feeling forgetful is disconcerting and can cause you to worry that it's a sign of your general decline. But the areas of the brain affecting memory and language are next to each other and studies show that learning a new language, writing a diary, doing your newspaper crossword and playing Scrabble are all good ways of sharpening your mind which will, in turn, boost your self-esteem. After a miserable divorce followed by a period of depression, a family friend felt as if she was sinking into mental decline. But then she remarried and, as her new husband had family in France, she decided to brush up her French. It was the intellectual challenge she needed, and really revived her self-esteem.

MIND GAMES

- Challenge yourself by reading different magazines, such as *The Times Literary Supplement* or *The New Yorker*.

- Play a category game, listing French cities, monarchs, classic cars, jazz musicians . . .

- List the 20 words you think are the most beautiful in the English language. Then list the ugliest, those that express joy, or those that are violent. Think of a new category each week.

- Try the A–Z game, where you list names (of, say, foreign capitals, boys' first names, composers or authors) in alphabetical order.

- Work at remembering your dreams. Learning to capture them on a daily basis is good memory-retrieval practice.

- Read: go to the library and read whatever takes your fancy – look for subjects new to you like history, genealogy or architecture, pick up a classic novel you always meant to read or delve into sci-fi or new experimental fiction.

- Do crosswords – they don't have to be hugely difficult but they're a good mental discipline.

- Play chess or bridge – apart from being mentally demanding, they're a good social activity.

Make new friends

The more you use your brain, the longer you'll retain your intellectual capabilities. As I mentioned above, becoming more mentally active is like becoming more physically active – it requires an overall change of approach, not just a quick fix. Doing a crossword every day is a good mental exercise, but it's no substitute for adopting a more mentally active approach to life. Achieving this means making new friends, developing new interests and exploring new challenges.

Humans are highly social animals with built-in social skills. But as with physical fitness, if you don't use your social skills, you will lose them. I've noted the importance of a healthy social life, and a recent study found that those with the most diverse social circle have a lower incidence of physical and mental health problems. Connecting with a variety of people strengthens our ability to cope with stress, and bolsters our immune systems.

Elsewhere in the book I've extolled the virtues of a clutter-free home, which can have benefits for your physical health (fewer allergic reactions) and psychological health (a clear desk always makes my brain feel fresh and ready for work). But clutter can extend into your social life too. How many people do you send Christmas cards to but never actually see or talk to during the year? If you like them, maybe you should call them on the phone, or meet up. Or maybe you should get out the red pen and cross them off the list!

Indulge yourself

Indulge in anti-ageing beauty treatments if they make you feel better about yourself. Older women often feel a sense of bereavement when they lose the looks they used to have. But most people who take the trouble to look their personal best, whatever age they are, are healthier as a result. When you feel good about yourself, you release neuropeptides, the so called 'molecules of emotion' which encourage health and well-being.

NEW YOU

Many successful people make a point of reinventing themselves every three or four years – by changing their career, altering their lifestyle or taking time out. You don't have to make radical changes, but you should keep moving forwards, taking the time to seek out new experiences, new people and new ideas. Life is about growing and learning; it's a process that never stops, and should become more interesting and enriching as we grow older and blend our previous experiences into new and more fulfilling versions of ourselves. Taking risks is also part of this ongoing process – a constantly renewed cycle of rejuvenation.

Battle with biology

Biological ageing can stem from two sources, which are technically known as intrinsic and extrinsic ageing. Intrinsic ageing is the ageing process programmed into our bodies which does not depend on external factors. This type of ageing involves the breakdown of normal cellular repair and renewal mechanisms, and is what limits your maximum possible lifespan to around a century. The rate at which this breakdown proceeds is determined by your genes; some people have genes for robust, long-lasting cellular repair machinery, and age more slowly than others (in intrinsic terms).

Extrinsic ageing is caused by 'external' factors – mainly sunlight and pollution (including toxins that you take in with food, water or smoke) and factors relating to nutritional quality. The key culprits here are free radicals, created by cellular metabolism and the action of ultraviolet light (in sunlight). Reactive compounds in pollution also introduce large quantities of damaging free radicals into your system. Free radicals bang about in your cells, damaging genetic material and cell walls and promoting degenerative changes. The more free radicals you're exposed to, the more damage they'll do to your cells, and the quicker you'll age.

According to one estimate, your body has to deal with around 10 trillion free radical 'hits' per day! Smoking, taking drugs and exposure to sunlight or pollution can increase this considerably (see below). Fortunately, your body is equipped with an array of defences against free radicals and their damaging effects, including molecules such as antioxidants that mop up the radicals, and other cellular machinery that repairs damaged DNA, proteins and so on. Intrinsic ageing causes the efficiency of these defences to decline, so that true ageing is largely caused by the interaction between extrinsic and intrinsic ageing.

Poor health habits accelerate biological ageing ahead of chronological age, so that you are more likely to suffer ill health and die early for your age. But good health habits can slow down your ageing so that, biologically speaking, you have the body of a much younger person.

To slow down the rate at which *your* body will age, you'll need to pay attention to the following.

Look after your skin

Since it's your skin that's most exposed to sunlight and external pollutants, it will bear the visible brunt of extrinsic ageing, making you look older before your time if you're unlucky. Free radicals created by UV light and pollutants damage collagen and elastic tissue, harm or kill cells in the skin growth layer and damage the cells that help maintain skin moisture and nourishment. At worst, skin can develop cancers.

While you can't (yet) change the genes that determine intrinsic ageing, you can exert some control over the factors that cause extrinsic ageing.

Most skin ageing is caused by sunlight, so as they say in Australia, slip, slop and slap – that is, slip on a shirt, slop on some sunscreen, and slap on a hat. (I wear a broadbrimmed cricket hat that keeps my whole face in the shade!) Always use SPF 15 or higher. Complete your ensemble with a pair of sunglasses.

Don't go out into the sun between 10am and 3pm, when the sun's UV rays are at their strongest. Be particularly careful in areas or countries with very strong sunshine (such as tropical areas) or where the ozone layer is thin, letting in more harmful UV rays (Australia/New Zealand or southern South America).

Don't be fooled into not bothering with sun protection by overcast or cloudy days – harmful UV rays can penetrate cloud cover and you could end up sustaining just as much damage. Definitely stay off sunbeds, and take extra care if you are fair-skinned.

Many vitamins and minerals act as antioxidants (which help with tissue repair), but the key ones for your skin are vitamins A, C and E. Having said which, the skin is often the last organ that gets a share of vitamins from your diet, so some specialists recommend topical supplementation – creams and serums containing vitamins A, C and E. Young-looking skin also owes a lot of its properties, such as elasticity, firmness, smoothness and suppleness, to its fat content – in particular, to the fatty acids that help to make strong, healthy cell walls and the sebum that helps the skin retain moisture and resist UV rays. Essential fatty acids are needed to make these skin fats, so ensuring a good dietary intake of fish, seeds and oils can help you keep your skin looking younger.

People often comment on the fact that my own skin looks so good. I put it down to a combination of lucky genes, a healthy diet and lifestyle, and the fact that I keep out of the sun. But I am also a firm believer in the benefits of exfoliation, which removes the dead cells on the outside and encourages cell renewal. So I start and end each day by splashing my face with warm water several times, then rubbing it over with a roughish towel. I use a little light moisturiser with at least SPF 15 sunblock, and the only make-up I use is mascara and lipstick (with no nasty chemicals).

Watch what you eat

I've devoted a big chunk of this book to food and eating habits – and in the long term, these become crucial factors in how well you age. Your diet influences your biological age in a big way, and can be a force for good or bad health. Junk food is an example of the latter. In my opinion, it's one of the curses of modern life, and should be avoided at all costs. By 'junk', I mean most refined prepared, processed foods. Both fast food outlets and supermarkets offer food that may be carrying a significant free radical content. Smoked and chargrilled foods are very good examples. Unfortunately, these make up a large percentage of what we eat these days. All too often, we're too busy to cook using raw materials, so we rely instead on ready-made foods, cooked up in factories. I want my sons to grow up cooking with fresh ingredients – so I have always encouraged them to cook at home, and my oldest boy, now 14, is such a dab hand in the kitchen I am still wondering what he did to a cottage pie recently to make the potato topping so delicious.

The problem with the fast food approach is what's hidden in the small print on the side of the packet – the truth about the extent to which processed food has been altered to make it longer lasting, easier to prepare and 'tastier'. Food is best eaten with as little done to it as possible, a principle that the food industry does not follow. Here are just a few of the evils of junk food:

- Most processed foods require chemical preservatives to extend their shelf life beyond the day or so that home-cooked foods remain nutritious.

- Colours and flavours are enhanced using chemicals.

- Large and unnecessary quantities of sugar and salt are added, along with saturated fat, to give the foods a good 'mouth feel'.

- Salt is even added to otherwise 'clean' bread, to stop it from going stale.

- Combining salt and sugar is a feature of some restaurant as well as factory cuisine, masking its presence through giving a fuller flavour to food.

- High fat content makes food taste more satisfying, but its presence is masked by the overall taste of the dish.

And that's just the stuff from the supermarket. The hamburgers, hot dogs, and so on available from fast food outlets fail enormously in the nutrition stakes. You have even less idea of what's gone into this type of food, as there are often no food labels to read. Because it's all processed, you can be sure it will contain more fat, salt, sugar and chemicals and free radicals than could possibly be considered 'healthy'.

Junk food will accelerate your biological ageing in one way or another. Additives such as colorants and preservatives can act as free radicals. Excess fats and sugars destabilise hormone production and contribute to cardiovascular ageing through overweight, high blood pressure and artherosclerosis. Salt has a damaging effect on many aspects of body function, particularly on blood pressure, which again stresses and prematurely ages the cardiovascular system, increasing the risk of heart disease and stroke.

Here's the vital message: give up fast foods, and work your way through the nutritional data on the back of all processed food packages that you are considering eating so you know how much fat, sugar and salt they contain. This will be a revelation, allowing you to select less damaging options – and eventually (in an ideal world, of course) wean yourself off processed foods altogether. Sorry to be so uncompromising about this, but paying a lot to get fat and die from heart disease just doesn't make sense to me!

Remember that it's those evil free radicals that do most of the damage to your skin and the rest of your body, so improving your diet to boost your intake of antioxidants (which help to mop up free radicals and limit the harm they can do) can help you stay younger.

Feed your brain too

A healthy diet will keep your brain in good working order too. Remember to eat oily fish such as sardines and mackerel, as the omega-3 fatty acids in them help keep the brain in good working order (as my granny always used to say: 'Fish makes good brains'). Don't let your healthy diet fall by the wayside just because you are elderly or living alone. You should also drink plenty of water to keep your brain hydrated.

There is a lot of talk currently about the benefits of certain nutritional supplements for the brain, such as gingko biloba. This is an emerging field and today's discoveries will, I am sure, be of huge benefit in the future. However, I urge people to avoid buying over-the-counter remedies without seeking good medical advice first.

ANOTHER GOOD REASON TO DRINK WATER!

Water has a major impact on your rate of biological ageing. Our bodies comprise around 65 per cent water, so it's hardly surprising that our vital processes depend upon the circulation of large amounts of it. Digestion, respiration, temperature control, organ function and waste removal are all dependent on water. As a result, your body is very sensitive to water deficiency, and that includes your skin. Good hydration is another defining characteristic of young-looking skin: a high moisture content helps to give skin its firmness, resilience and smoothness. When skin dries out, the bonds between its elastic fibres break more easily and its cells become more vulnerable. Drinking a lot of water can help to prevent this – as can avoiding substances that dehydrate you (such as caffeine in tea, coffee and soft drinks). Water also helps to flush toxins out of your system, which again benefits the skin.

Change your lifestyle

If I took 'before' and 'after' photos of my patients, you'd see noticeable changes in their appearance – and also in their attitudes, which can be quite remarkable. This is great for me, as well, as it reinforces the basic philosophy by which I work.

You can make a big difference to your biological age and your skin in particular by avoiding the bad habits that increase your exposure to free radicals and dehydrate your skin. Here are some vital tips:

- Cigarettes: smoking is top of the list of things to avoid (see overleaf) – according to one estimate, each drag of a cigarette exposes you to 3 trillion free radical 'hits'! Smoking narrows blood vessels and impairs circulation to your skin. It also leaches vitamins out of your system (such as vitamin C), and degrades its elasticity. As well as the other warnings on a cigarette packet I think there should be the message: 'Smoking makes you look old.'

- Drink: alcohol dehydrates you.

- Recreational drugs may flood your system with free radicals and often lead to dehydration.

- Environmental pollution (including cigarette smoke) generates free radicals. I have discussed measures you can take to counteract this in Chapter 8.

- Staying up late tends to drain your reserves. I have many successful models as patients who, despite the public perception of their non-stop partying, find they have to go to bed by 11pm if they want to stay in work. Staying up all night, drinking and smoking shows in your skin. After the age of 25, this is even more obvious.

- The bigger picture: as you've probably worked out, many of these factors go hand in hand – a late-night lifestyle of alcohol, cigarettes and drugs is likely to prematurely age you. A saintly lifestyle of early nights, abstinence and pure air and water will keep you looking young for longer. Having said that, I am, as you'll have gathered, not puritanical and don't expect my patients to be. My aim is to get people to think about what they are doing and the rationale for making changes.

HOW TO GIVE UP SMOKING

Nicotine is psychologically and physically addictive because smoking is a social, everyday, routine habit that is part of the lifestyle of so many people. There has been a huge increase in smoking among women, coinciding with an increase in binge drinking. Lung cancer, which is directly linked to smoking, is one of the biggest killers of women and has now outstripped breast cancer. What's more, smoking causes wrinkles and lines around the mouth and eyes, together with dull skin – surely enough to put most people off.

When people start smoking, the first few cigarettes make them nauseated and dizzy as their systems react to nicotine's toxic effects. But the body adjusts with frightening speed and the drug quickly becomes enjoyable.

Unfortunately, nicotine's enjoyable effects are in themselves damaging.

Nicotine stimulates the adrenal glands to pump adrenalin into the bloodstream, raising blood pressure and heart rate and increasing gastrointestinal activity. This physiological reaction is similar to the so-called 'fight or flight' response, which the body uses to ready itself for action when in danger.

Nicotine in small quantities stimulates the brain, giving a sense of well-being in the same way caffeine does, but there is a depressive counter-reaction from nicotine in larger quantities. At the same time, nicotine is also a muscle relaxant, acting in opposition to the other physical reactions. The chemical effects of nicotine are very damaging, particularly as smokers put themselves through this harmful exposure many times each day. In larger amounts, such as in people who smoke really heavily, nicotine acts as a sedative.

The process of giving up smoking can be somewhat unpleasant, as the body struggles to re-establish its normal metabolism after years of abuse. Giving up is often accompanied by 'cold turkey' symptoms such as tension and extreme irritability. Smoking artificially boosts blood sugar levels, but when people stop there is a counter-reaction that causes low levels of blood sugar. This makes them feel weak and can lead to overeating and weight gain. Former smokers may cough more after stopping smoking, as a healthy lining grows back in their lungs. This will settle down in time, though.

For many, however, it's the cultural aspect of smoking that presents the greatest obstacle to giving up. As I tell my patients, it's comparatively easy to quit smoking but there may be more work to do before you transform yourself into a non-smoker. Smoking creates its own social dimension, an identity that is very hard to shake off. Many people 'quit' but still feel like smokers, and so fall back under stress or a social situation that feels more comfortable with a cigarette in one hand and a glass of wine in the other.

The banning of smoking in public places, offices, restaurants and bars will make it far easier for people to give up, and will also remove that most unreasonable and irresponsible of risks to the health of others – passive smoking.

Look Forward

- The rate at which you will age is influenced by your genes – but also by how well you look after yourself.

- Don't delay thinking about how you will age. It is happening from your twenties – long before you will see the damage. This is when you should be starting to take preventative measures.

- There are no shortcuts! A healthy diet and lifestyle are the best ways to stay looking and feeling young.

To conclude

One of the key concepts of naturopathy is that you stand a better chance of living a healthy life if you take control of it instead of letting your doctor make every decision for you. It's something we should all seek to do. But becoming a healthier person is not something you can put a deadline on. It is an ongoing process. Maintaining optimum health involves not just consolidating changes you've already made, but constantly learning new ways to enhance and change your lifestyle – new forms of exercise, new elements you can add to your diet, new ways to get in touch with your creativity and your environment.

Variety is essential; you don't want to get stuck in a rut, doing the same things every day, because you'll quickly lose enthusiasm and motivation. Programmes should be adapted to fit your personal circumstances, but of course circumstances change, so your programmes should be flexible. Don't junk a whole exercise programme just because you missed one day of it. If you move house and are no longer near a gym, think about taking up a different form of exercise – walking or running, for instance. There is always something you can do to fit in with your current lifestyle. For example, women who have just had a baby can go for long walks with the buggy, and those who are housebound can exercise in the home.

Total health isn't just about losing a stone or being able to run a marathon; it's more to do with making fundamental changes to your attitude and your outlook. In other words, the most important daily essential isn't a routine, a diet or a programme, but a reaffirmation of your positive healthy-living aspirations and values – saying to yourself, 'Every day, in every way, I am going to work towards the best, healthiest, happiest life possible.'

Set yourself ambitious but attainable long-term goals and break them down into intermediate targets. Then break these down further until you arrive at a series of day-to-day goals which are challenging but not unrealistic.

Recognise when you've attained one of your goals, and reward yourself for doing so, even if this simply means patting yourself on the back. Recognising your achievements helps to boost your self-esteem and self-confidence, making it much easier to sustain the motivation to follow and complete a programme.

Setting intermediate goals that also enhance the health of your lifestyle is a brilliant way to sustain day-to-day changes. Goals can be in any area of your life, but it makes sense to set ones that combine different elements, such as getting fit to do something active that involves charity or community work.

Good examples might include training to run a marathon to raise funds for charity, or for a walking holiday in Nepal; undertaking a series of sponsored walks to raise funds to send yourself on a volunteer programme to an exotic place; studying for an exam or qualification that will help you travel or explore – such as a language or scuba diving; or working towards a coaching or instructor's badge so that you can teach a sport or martial art in a local youth centre. All these examples combine the attributes of being multifunctional, ambitious, worthwhile and fun.

THE 10 HEALTHY HABITS OF PEOPLE WHO LIVE NATUROPATHICALLY

1. **Know your body** – recognise what's normal for you, and what's not. Watch your body closely for symptoms of all kinds. It is trying to tell you things all the time, and it is down to you to listen to what it's saying!

2. **Take charge of your health** – see your GP as someone you can trust to help you address problems you have identified. As I said early in the book, there are many passive patients who believe their problems are

their doctors' to solve. A healthier approach is to see your doctor as a partner who can give you the wherewithal (the diagnosis, the referral, the management options) to help yourself.

3. **Eat a fresh and varied diet** based around fish, a range of grains and pulses, and organic vegetables. Use your diet diary. You will see how well you feel when you have been eating a good, fresh whole food diet, and how your body misses this when a holiday or business trip prevents you from eating what has now become normal for you.

4. **Eat regularly and moderately**: 'Everything in moderation,' as Socrates said. You will soon get to know how your body responds to a few days of overindulgence, or a lazy period when you just can't be bothered to eat properly.

5. **Enjoy an active life**, in which exercise has a natural place. There's no such thing as 'no time for exercise'. If you don't believe me, take another look at my own exercise diary on page 147 to see how I fit physical wellbeing into my very busy daily life.

6. **Make the most of your surroundings**. Enjoy fresh air and sunlight. Take 'a walk with a view' – looking at vistas and horizons is good for the mind. Feel the early morning or late night dew on your bare feet. These things are free – and they can have a dramatic effect on your psychological wellbeing.

7. **Sleep well and get plenty of rest**. This is a not to be underrated – and crucial to good health. See page 247 for my tips.

8. **Have a good work–life balance**. Make sure you have time to 'stand and stare'. Don't be one of the many people I see each week who say, 'Where did my twenties go?' 'What happened to my thirties?' 'Why don't I remember my children growing up?' Or 'One minute I was looking forward to my life; the next I could only look back . . . '

9. **Trust your intuition**. As I said in the introduction to this book, before we had all the medical tests doctors use these days, physicians

trusted instinct and intuition. Likewise, you should always follow your own instinct and seek help if you have concerns.

10. **Be happy** . . . I know you can't be happy to order, but I hope that in using the advice from this book you will be able to take control of your life, and find ways in which you can find the fulfilment you deserve.

And finally . . .

Are you feeling inspired? Or daunted? Don't worry: Rome wasn't built in a day. Don't try too much at once, and accept that there will be backsliding into old habits, moments of weakness, and times when you will be fed up with the whole 'being healthy' thing. Don't be hard on yourself, which is self-defeating. But do press on with doing your best to implement changes in your life so that you can reap the benefits. Once you do start to feel improvements to how you feel, and you start to see the changes to your waistline and all the other measurables, you will be more motivated to continue – and the improvements will come more easily. Remember that the goal is to achieve a plateau of good health, harmony and wellbeing – and this is remarkably difficult to lose once you have reached it.

But, if you can do just one thing to improve your health, give up smoking . . . and, please don't start again. Or, if you backslide, have the perseverance to give it up as many times as it takes until you have finally given up completely.

After this, the most important requirement is that you enjoy your life. Healthy living isn't about Puritanism and stoic self-denial. You can enjoy everything in moderation, but by no means will this lessen your enjoyment. Trust me, it's a great life!

Resources

Alexander Technique

For details of local organisations and practitioner lists:

Alexander Technique International
www.alextechnique.cib.net

Allergy

To find out more about specific allergies, treatments, news and anti-allergy products:

Allergy UK
www.allergyfoundation.com

AESSRA: Allergy and Environmental Sensitivity Support and Research Organisation, Australia
home.vicnet.net.au/~aessra

Allergy/Asthma Information Association, Canada
www.aaia.ca

Allergy New Zealand Inc
www.allergy.org.nz

Allergy Society of South Africa
www.allergysa.org

Breast Cancer

For support and information:

Breast Cancer Care
www.breastcancercare.org.uk

National Breast Cancer Centre Australia
www.nbcc.au

Canadian Breast Cancer Network
www.cbcn.ca

New Zealand Breast Cancer Foundation
www.breast.co.nz

Cancer

For information on other cancers and cancer organisations:

Cancerbacup UK
www.cancerbacup.org.uk

Cancer Research UK
www.cancerresearchuk.org

Cancer Council Australia
www.cancer.org.au

Cure Cancer Australia
www.curecancer.org.au

Canadian Cancer Society
www.cancer.ca

Cancer Society of New Zealand
www.cancernz.org.nz

Cancer Association of South Africa
cansa.org.za

Digestive Disorders

The following has good information pages on a range of digestive disorders:

Digestive Disorders Foundation
www.digestivedisorders.org.uk

Food Standards

The following has useful information pages on healthy diet and a Body Mass Index calculator:

Food Standards Agency UK
www.foodstandards.gov.uk

Heart Disease

For details of support groups, news and information on treating and preventing heart disease:

British Heart Foundation
www.bhf.org.uk

National Heart Foundation of Australia
www.heartfoundation.com.au

The Heart and Stroke Foundation of Canada
www.heartandstroke.ca

National Heart Foundation of New Zealand
www.heartfoundation.org.nz

Heart Foundation of South Africa
www.afronets.org

Meditation

For step-by-step advice on learning to meditate:

World Wide Online Meditation Centre
www.meditationcentre.com

Naturopathy

To find a naturopathic practitioner:

General Council and Register of Naturopaths
www.naturopathy.org.uk

Australian Naturopathy Network
www.ann.com.au

The Canadian Association of Naturopathic Physicians
www.naturopathic.org/find/canada.html

New Zealand Society of Naturopaths Inc
www.naturopath.org.nz

Nutrition

For up-to-date news and advice on specific aspects of nutrition:

British Nutrition Foundation
www.nutrition.org.uk

Nutrition Australia
www.nutritionaustralia.org

The National Institute of Nutrition, Canada
www.nin.ca

Nutrition Society of New Zealand
www.nutritionsociety.ac.nz

Nutrition Society of South Africa
www.nutritionsociety.co.za

Pilates

For details of Pilates teachers, exercise programmes, and products:

Pilates Foundation UK
www.pilatesfoundation.com

Australian Pilates Method Association
www.bodycontrol.co.uk/australia.html

Pilates Body Control (South Africa)
www.bodycontrol.co.uk/south.africa.html

Vegan Societies

Useful advice for vegans:

Vegan Society of Australia
www.veganaustralia.org

Vegans in Canada/USA
www.vegans.com

Vegan Society of New Zealand
www.veganz.pl.net/

Vegans in South Africa
home.intekom.com/animals/orgs/visa/

Vegetarianism

For advice on vegetarianism:

Vegetarian Society
UK www.vegsoc.org

Australian Vegetarian Society
www.veg-soc.org

The Toronto Vegetarian Association
www.veg.ca

New Zealand Vegetarian Society
www.ivu.org/nzvs

Water Purifiers

The following are stockists of water purifiers for the home:

Healthy House, UK
www.healthy-house.co.uk

Purifiers Australia
www.purifiersaustralia.com.au/

Purifiers in Canada/USA
www.generalecology.com/qa.htm

H2O Water Purifiers, South Africa
www.h2o.co.za/

Yoga

For advice on postures, books, tapes and links with other yoga organisations:

www.yogasite.com

Index

80:20 rule (Pareto Principle) 260

abdominal pain 187–8, 193
abortion 219
acid reflux 187–8, 193
acne 123, 124
Addenbrookes Diet 74–8
additives 63, 73, 138
adrenalin 285
aerobic exercise 145–6, 150–6
    boredom with 156
    cautions regarding 154–5
    definition 145
    slow start rule 155–6
    types 151–4
age, physiological/chronological 124
age-related macular degeneration 32
ageing 225–6, 270–86
    battling biology 278–85
    and diet 280–3
    extrinsic 278–9
    intrinsic 278, 279
    and lifestyle 283–4
    psychological issues 275–8
    skin 279–80
air filters 104, 110, 112
alcohol consumption 283

alcoholic content 39–40
    binge drinking 29, 40
    effects of 40, 41
    recommended levels 39–40
    signs of heavy 124
Alexander, F. Matthias 168
Alexander Technique 163, 168
alkaline broth 136
allergens 96–7, 99
allergic reactions 68
allergies 12
    see also hay fever
    biochemical basis 22
    to cosmetics 109, 121–2
    definition 68
    food 52, 63, 68–78
    symptoms 69–74, 124, 125
allergy diaries 70, 73–4, 75
altruism 232
aluminium 113
ambition 256–7
amino acids, essential 30
amylase 85
anaemia 58–9, 140, 192, 193
anaerobic exercise 145
anal region, soiling 131
anaphylactic shock 68